LFA He

T'ai Chi N

Movements 1 – 1ɔ∪

Explained in an easy to follow format

By Sheila Dickinson
President of the LFA Health Arts

Benefits:-
Helps to improve balance and co-ordination
Helps to improve joint mobility and reflexes
Eases Stress
Provides Relaxation

Printed and published in Great Britain by

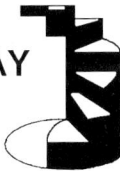

STAIRWAY
DISTRIBUTION
LTD.

P 0 BOX 19,
HEDON,
HULL
HU12 8YR

First Published 2003

Published by Stairway Distribution Limited
PO Box 19, Hedon. Hull. HU12 8YR
www.leefamilyarts.com

Please consult your Doctor before taking part in the following exercise programme.
The LFA and Stairway Distribution Ltd disclaim any liability for loss or injury in connection with the advice and exercises included in this book.

Acknowledgements

To the past Masters of our Arts - we offer our sincere
thanks!

THE LFA T'AI CHI LIBRARY

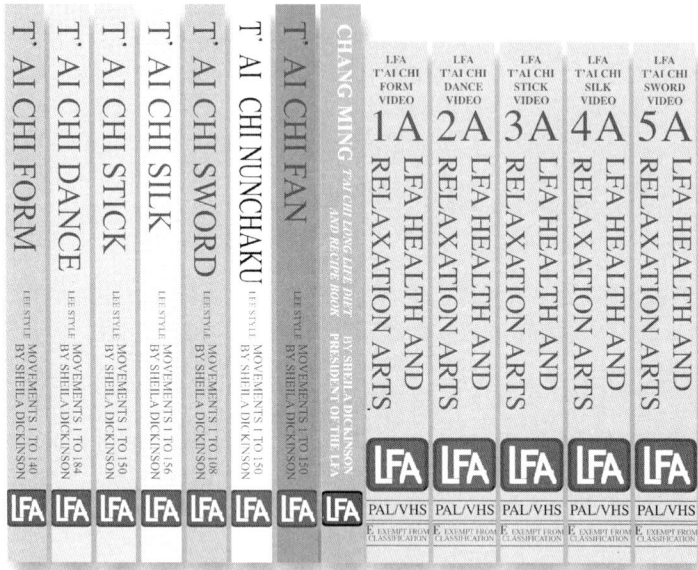

T'AI CHI FORM — LEE STYLE — MOVEMENTS 1 TO 140 BY SHEILA DICKINSON — LFA

T'AI CHI DANCE — LEE STYLE — MOVEMENTS 1 TO 184 BY SHEILA DICKINSON — LFA

T'AI CHI STICK — LEE STYLE — MOVEMENTS 1 TO 150 BY SHEILA DICKINSON — LFA

T'AI CHI SILK — LEE STYLE — MOVEMENTS 1 TO 56 BY SHEILA DICKINSON — LFA

T'AI CHI SWORD — LEE STYLE — MOVEMENTS 1 TO 150 BY SHEILA DICKINSON — LFA

T'AI CHI NUNCHAKU — LEE STYLE — MOVEMENTS 1 TO 108 BY SHEILA DICKINSON — LFA

T'AI CHI FAN — LEE STYLE — MOVEMENTS 1 TO 150 BY SHEILA DICKINSON — LFA

CHANG MING — T'AI CHI LONG LIFE DIET AND RECIPE BOOK — BY SHEILA DICKINSON PRESIDENT OF THE LFA — LFA

LFA T'AI CHI FORM VIDEO	LFA T'AI CHI DANCE VIDEO	LFA T'AI CHI STICK VIDEO	LFA T'AI CHI SILK VIDEO	LFA T'AI CHI SWORD VIDEO
1A	2A	3A	4A	5A
LFA HEALTH AND RELAXATION ARTS	LFA HEALTH AND RELAXATION ARTS	LFA HEALTH AND RELAXATION ARTS	LFA HEALTH AND RELAXATION ARTS	LFA HEALTH AND RELAXATION ARTS
LFA	LFA	LFA	LFA	LFA
PAL/VHS	PAL/VHS	PAL/VHS	PAL/VHS	PAL/VHS
E EXEMPT FROM CLASSIFICATION	E EXEMPT FROM CLASSIFICATION	E EXEMPT FROM CLASSIFICATION	E EXEMPT FROM CLASSIFICATION	E EXEMPT FROM CLASSIFICATION

All of the above Books and Videos are available from:-
Stairway Distribution Limited
PO Box 19
Hedon
HU12 8YR
Tel/Fax 01482 896063

You may also order from our Websites, please visit:
www.leefamilyarts.com   www.lfataichi.com

CONTENTS

Foreword

Welcome to the Lee Family Arts T'ai Chi Nunchaku Set. Please note, I have used the same foreword in each of my books in order that I can pay tribute to my late Grand Master, Chee Soo.

My position as President of the Lee Family Arts started in January 1995. Since that time, I have had the privilege to guide my fellow instructors in all aspects of LFA T'ai Chi, and I have worked hard to reach as many people as possible, so that everyone may gain from the many health benefits of our Arts.

I would not be writing this book today without the guidance and patience of my late Grand Master Chee Soo, who spent most of his life teaching the Lee Family Arts. Chee Soo is in my thoughts constantly and I offer my sincere thanks for receiving the benefit of his wisdom and understanding.

Chee Soo wrote five books published by the Aquarian Press, sadly at the time of writing only one title remains in print today 'The Chinese Art of T'ai Chi Ch'uan'. In this book he traces the history of the Lee Style back to Ho-Hsieh Lee circa 1,000BC. It is stated that the Lee Family have always been Taoists and that the Lee Style is a Yin and Yang style, this means that everything within it is in complete balance and harmony.

1

Chee Soo occasionally spoke of his own Grand Master, Chan Kam Lee and told of how they had met during 1934 in Hyde Park in London. In those days there were very few Oriental people in London and the two became friends. It was a friendship that would change Chee Soo's life forever. After Chan Kam Lee's death, Chee Soo dedicated himself to maintaining the knowledge and wisdom he had learnt from Chan Kam Lee.

While staying with my family and my self, Chee Soo talked to me about the future of the Lee Family Arts and the direction he wished them to take. On Monday the 16th May 1994 Chee Soo asked me to give him my word that I would not let the Lee Family Arts die.

Sadly Chee Soo died on the 29th August 1994.

It is with the greatest respect to Chee Soo that I offer my own writings and understanding of the lessons he taught me.

The names of Instructors who have trained, qualified and still maintain their own training can be obtained from the Lee Family Arts official register of qualified instructors. The LFA can only vouch for the quality and content of that which is taught within an official LFA registered class.

The Lee Family Arts have been tried and tested for

thousands of years before we were born. The people who teach them are merely caretakers, who have the privilege of maintaining the Arts, and witnessing them helping others.

This book teaches you the first one hundred and fifty movements of the LFA T'ai Chi Nunchaku Set. There are two hundred and seventy movements in total and these latter movements will be explained in further publications. The Lee Family Arts will always be known as a Family Art and it is a family which grows in numbers daily. In concluding, I would like to say a very special welcome to you!

'The Wisdom of Our Arts'

The Ancient Masters were very particular regarding to whom they passed their knowledge on to. Their priceless information had been handed down from generation to generation, over many centuries. Chan Kam Lee, who brought the Lee Style out of China in the nineteen thirties, was no exception. The only person who knew the true knowledge and depth of his teachings was his adopted nephew called Chee Soo. If you have studied all of the movements written in the LFA series of books, I am sure that you would not think that you have the complete understanding of our Arts. This can only be passed on to you as you evolve to such a level of understanding that you know you are capable of being able to accept the great gift of knowledge which is available to you. This can be obtained by people who give the time and dedication to their training. It is up to everyone to prove their willingness to help others, and above all follow the instructions of the Master who holds the essence of the LFA Health Arts. The LFA do not boast of many secrets, we teach you to practise the movements of our Arts. The movements work, how much time you allocate to practising our Arts it is up to you. We can guide you to obtain the true understanding which comes from within each of us.

Many different classes offer to teach you the movements of T'ai Chi, only classes which are registered within the LFA Association can teach you the depth of the movements within our Arts, only the Master can guide you to the deepest level of understanding. We offer day courses and workshops throughout the year, giving you the opportunity to develop the depth of understanding of LFA T'ai Chi, which is within the reach of everyone.

Your inner power is something you should feel, through the dedicated practise of our movements.

This book teaches you the first one hundred and fifty movements of our Nunchaku set. Originally the nunchaku was used within the self-defence side of our Arts. However it is considered to be of great value to people of all ages as the flowing movements, help to improve everyone's balance, co-ordination and reflexes. It brings a smile to the faces of all practitioners as they learn to improve their skills in this beautiful flowing sequence of movements.

Chan Kam Lee advised that everyone should lead a clean and pure life in mind, body and spirit, and always follow they way of the Tao. He also recommended that you should first control your mind, then your spirit and then your body. A list of his eight golden rules as laid down in 1931 can be found in Chee Soo's book 'The Taoist Art of Feng Shou'.

What is Tao Yin?

Tao Yin is Taoist respiration therapy. This kind of breathing started long ago in China and was adopted by the Taoists who realised that this type of breathing was essential to good health. In addition, they also realised that everything needs to breathe in order to live; Chee Soo was often quoted as saying 'breath is life'.

The Ancient Taoists experimented with air to find the true benefits which it could give, both to the physical and spiritual side of their lives.

The basic foundation of this art came with the 'Sons of Reflected Light'. The Sons of Reflected Light were reputed to be a sect of people over seven feet tall, who wore a type of clothing never before seen in China. Where they came from was unknown and even until this day no one seems to know the true answer. Throughout their stay in China, they taught many skills far in advance of their day and some in advance of today. Great effort has been taken by Taoists over the centuries to carry on their work. Sadly, nothing was written down and some of the skills have been lost with the passing of time. However, the most important of all the skills was an array of health arts. It is the aim of the LFA to preserve these Arts and teach them to others so that everyone may benefit. Remember that our Arts have been kept alive by the Taoists for many thousands of years.

Chee explained that they aimed for two main objectives, firstly to maintain a longer life here on earth and secondly to achieve a stronger spiritual link with the Supreme Spirit. They tried to accept each day as it came, by understanding and abiding with the laws of the universe and the Tao.

Tao Yin breathing is used within our breathing exercises and K'ai Men exercises which are taught in all of the LFA classes, day courses, Easter Courses, and summer courses. We will always help you to reap the benefits of the centuries of training and understanding which have gone before.

Taoist Walk

In the LFA we teach the importance of the Taoist Walk, it is included in every book written in this series. The principles of the Taoist Walk apply to all aspects of our health. For example, when the Taoist Walk is harmonised with our specialised breathing exercises and hand movements (which are taught within our classes), it helps to boost the vigour of the immune system. Another exercise, when combined with the Taoist Walk, benefits the heart. We also have specialised movements which, while helping to rejuvenate different parts of the body, also provide quite dynamic self defence techniques.

Taoist Walk

The Taoist walk is an extremely important part of the LFA health training because it moves the weight from one leg to another in a special and subtle way. Not only is one leg working while the other one rests, but the working leg is the Yang leg and the resting leg is the Yin leg.

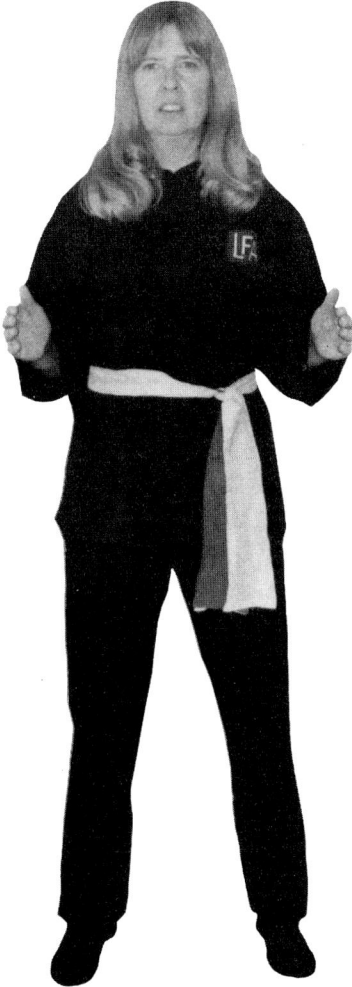

The weight is moved from one leg to the other <u>before</u> you try to alter the position of your foot.

Start with your feet slightly wider than shoulder width apart, toes pointing forwards. Both hands are held at waist height with the palms facing each other.

1/ Drift your weight across to your right side, your right knee bends, your hips and your bottom move across to the right side.

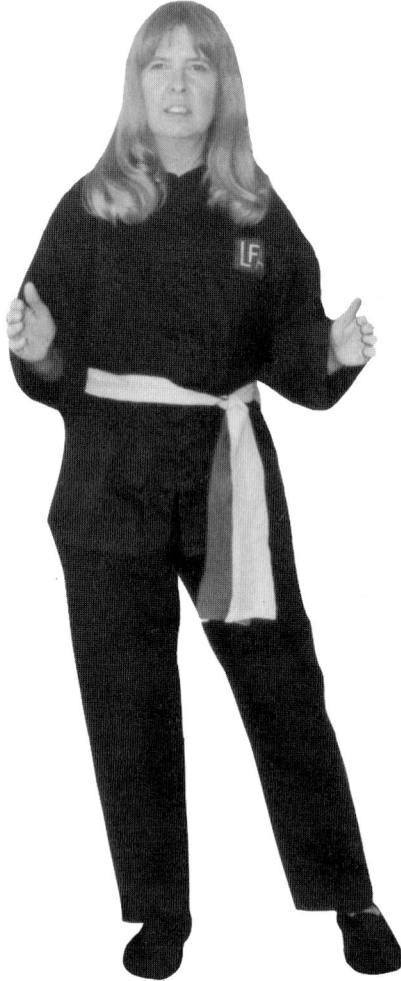

2/ Now take a very small step forwards with your left foot, placing your heel down first. Allow your left knee to bend, move your hips and bottom across to the left. Keep your right leg straight, do not lock your right knee.

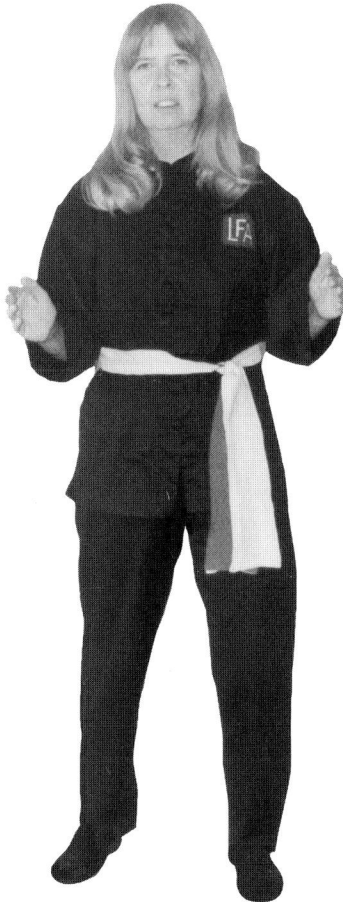

Practise walking across the room in this manner. People suffering from back, hip, knee and ankle problems, reap great benefits from practising the Taoist Walk.

We use the Taoist Walk in all of our form sets. With practise it can be incorporated into your every day walk (so that it is undetectable), only you will know the benefits you are receiving each time you place one foot in front of the other.

The Taoist Walk helps to move your Chi energy into the lower part of your body. In the West we tend to carry a lot of energy congestion around the pelvic area, this stagnation leads to the above mentioned problems. So it is a good idea to learn to walk the Taoist Way.

Please try it for yourself, especially if you wake up in the morning feeling stiff, a few minutes practising the Taoist Walk could help to make you feel like a new man or woman.

Etiquette

The etiquette is something which has been handed down through the centuries along with the T'ai Chi, I personally feel it represents a respect for the Arts we are practising and the ancient Masters to whom we owe so much.

When entering or leaving a training hall, the student should bow to the room. This bow consists of bending forwards from the waist, at the same time, both palms rest on your thighs.

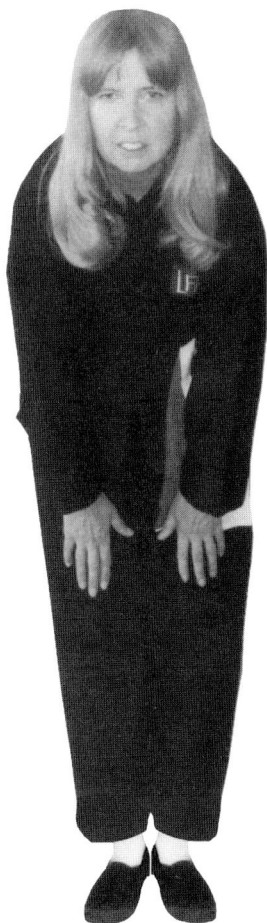

If you arrive after a class has already started you should walk round to the front of the hall, bow to the person taking the class and wait for them to bow to you in return (using the bow explained below). At the beginning of a class the bow consists of placing your right arm on top of your left in front of your body, your right palm faces down, and your left palm faces up.

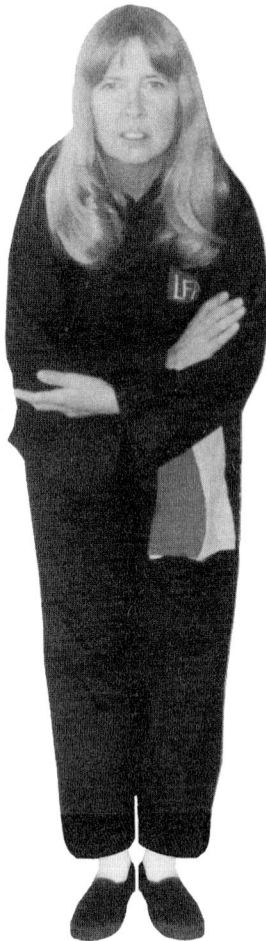

When training with a partner you should both bow to each other at the start and finish (using the same bow as when entering and leaving the training room).

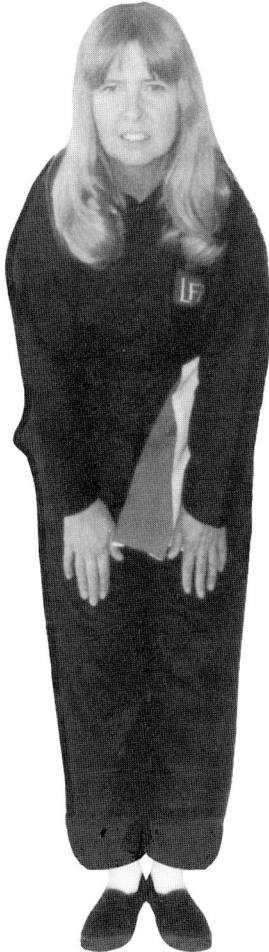

If an instructor offers you guidance with your training, you should bow to them after they have finished teaching you, (again using the bow for entering and leaving the training room).

LFA T'ai Chi Nunchaku Set

Practising our Nunchaku sets brings a smile to the face of every student. The movements are fun to learn and they improve your balance, co-ordination and reflexes.

In our classes we use foam safety cord nunchakus as they are light and easy to hold. Students from twelve years of age to people over eighty years young enjoy the many health benefits to be gained.

The movements are first learnt mechanically, once you have mastered this first stage it is time to harmonise your breathing with your movements.

Your hand and feet movements plus your breathing should all start and finish at the same time. With practise you will begin to feel the true essence contained within our Nunchaku set.

Do not try and rush the process, take the time to feel what is going on inside your body. Advanced students are eventually taught to practise the Nunchaku set with their eyes closed as this helps to improve the individual's awareness. The Nunchaku set is made up of many layers. Master one level only to find another waiting underneath.

It is the sheer depth of knowledge contained within the Lee Family Arts that makes it so interesting.

LFA T'ai Chi Stances

Although you may be eager to press on and learn the beneficial movements of our Nunchaku set, it is important that you take the time to familiarise yourself with our stances.

First become familiar with their names, next check the position of your feet. It is important that you have the correct weight distribution without any strain on your body. If you attend a weekly class, your instructor will be able to advise you. However if you are unable to attend classes, I suggest you stand in front of a mirror to help you to achieve a good posture.

It is important to remember that our feet provide our roots, without which we will fall over. Take the time to move from one stance to another applying the Taoist Walk, only in this way will you reap the full benefits which are on offer to everyone.

In these early stages of your training, try to feel what is happening to the muscles of your body as you move slowly from one position to the next. Later on you will appreciate a far greater depth to the movements you are practising. The person who takes their time and learns patience will eventually achieve a far greater benefit from our Arts than the person who rushes on believing they know all the movements of a particular form set. Judging your progress by numbers is very much a western concept, the LFA are purely interested in improving the quality of your life. There is no time limit, or pressure applied to your journey with us. Enjoy learning and practising our Arts, and find the path to a different way of living.

Bear Stance

Bear stance is achieved by standing with your feet shoulder width apart. Your body should be relaxed with no tension. Both of your arms should be hanging loosely by your sides. You should be looking straight ahead.

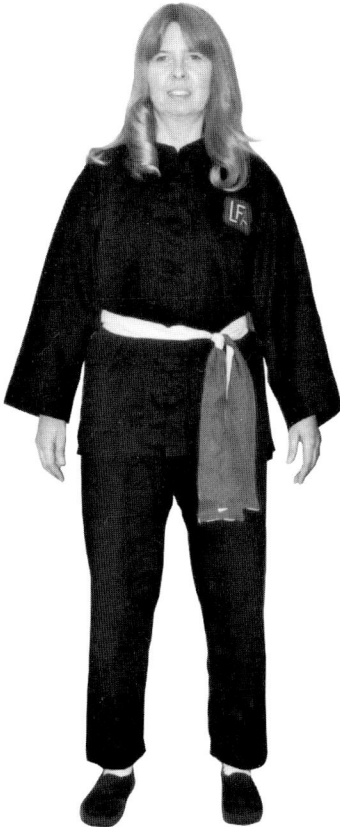

We use Bear stance at the beginning of all of our sets, when we adopt the 'Prepare' position.

Bee Stance

Bee stance is achieved, by standing with both heels together, your toes are pointing slightly outwards with both knees bent. Both arms hang loosely by your sides. Your eyes should be looking straight ahead.

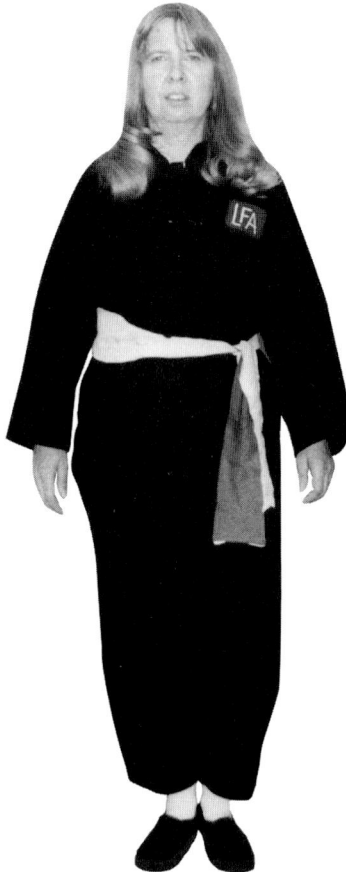

Cat Stance

To achieve a Right Cat stance, the left leg is bent at the knee, the heel is raised on your right foot. The ball of the right foot rests lightly on the floor with eighty percent of your weight on your left leg.

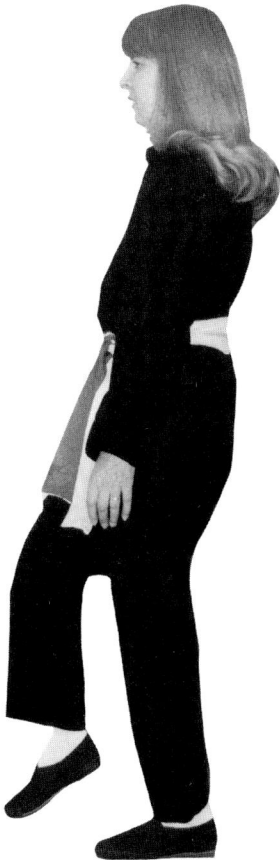

To achieve a Left Cat stance, the right leg is bent at the knee, the heel is raised on your left foot. The ball of your left foot rests lightly on the floor with eighty percent of your weight on your right leg.

Chicken Stance

To achieve a Right Chicken stance turn ninety degrees to your right. Now place most of your weight onto your right leg (bending the knee). Next bend and lower your left knee towards the floor. This is quite a strong stance, it is important that you listen to your own body and do not strain.

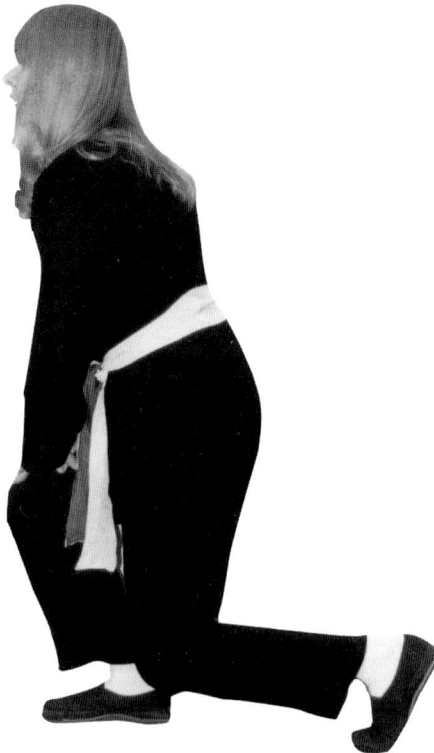

To achieve a Left Chicken stance turn ninety degrees to your left. Now place most of your weight onto your left leg (bending the knee). Next bend and lower your right knee towards the floor. This is quite a strong stance, again it is important that you listen to your own body and do not strain.

Crane Stance

To achieve a Right Crane stance move your weight onto your left leg (bending your left knee slightly to aid your balance). At the same time raise your right leg (bending your right knee) until your thigh is parallel with the floor. Students who have difficulty balancing should use a Cat stance for movements which require one leg to be lifted off the floor.

To achieve a Left Crane stance take your weight onto your right leg (bending your right knee slightly to aid your balance). At the same time raise your left leg (bending your left knee) until your thigh is parallel with the floor.

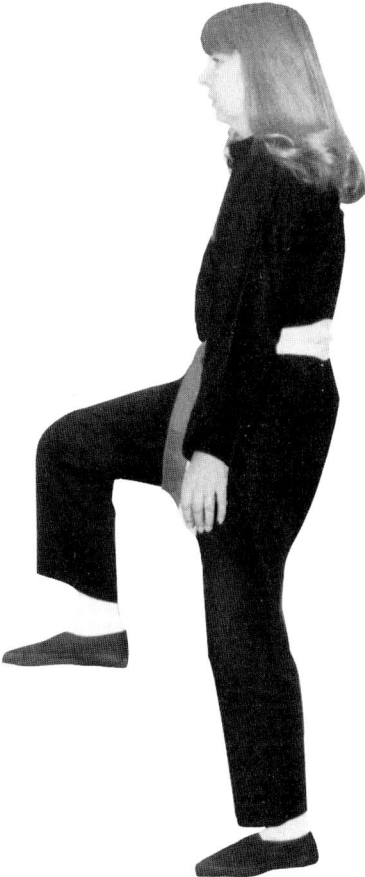

Crossed Legs Stance

To achieve Right Crossed Legs stance, bend your left knee slightly. Now cross your right leg in front of and slightly beyond your left leg, raise the heel of your right foot.

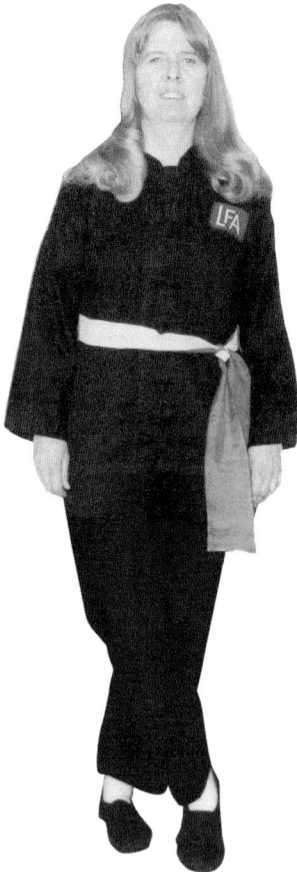

To achieve Left Crossed Legs stance, bend your right knee slightly. Now cross your left leg in front of and slightly beyond your right leg, raise the heel of your left foot.

Dog Stance

To achieve Right Dog stance move your weight onto your left leg (bending your knee slightly to aid your balance). At the same time extend and raise your right leg forwards, your leg should be at a height which is comfortable to you without strain.

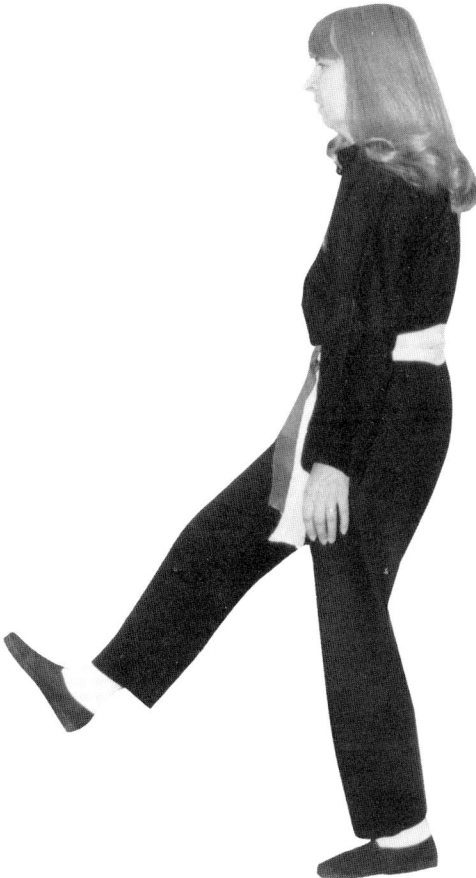

To achieve Left Dog stance, move your weight onto your right leg (bending your knee slightly to aid your balance). At the same time extend and raise your left leg forwards.

Dragon Stance

To achieve a Right Dragon stance step forwards from either a Bear or an Eagle stance. It is important not to overstep, make sure you have a good gap (width ways) between your feet.

Drift your weight over to your right side, so that the weight is spread between your right hip, knee and ankle. Eighty percent of your weight should be on your right leg, your left leg should be straight although not locked.

To achieve a Left Dragon stance, follow the same procedure as above this time stepping forward with your left leg.

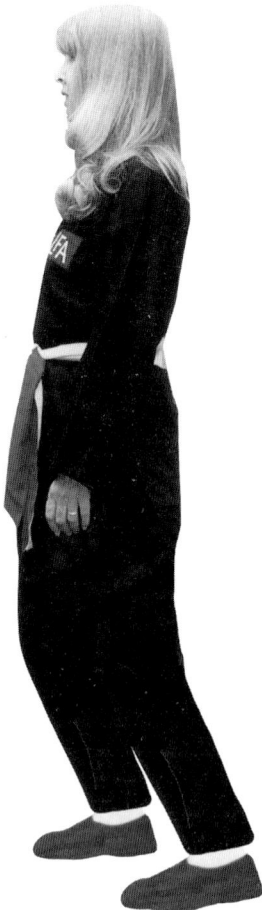

Duck Stance

To achieve a Right Duck stance from Eagle stance, step behind with your left foot, placing your heel down first. Now drift your weight onto your left leg (bending your knee), your right leg should be straight, although not locked.

To achieve a Left Duck stance from Eagle stance, step back with your right foot, placing your heel down first. Now drift your weight onto your right leg (bending your knee), your left leg should be straight, although not locked.

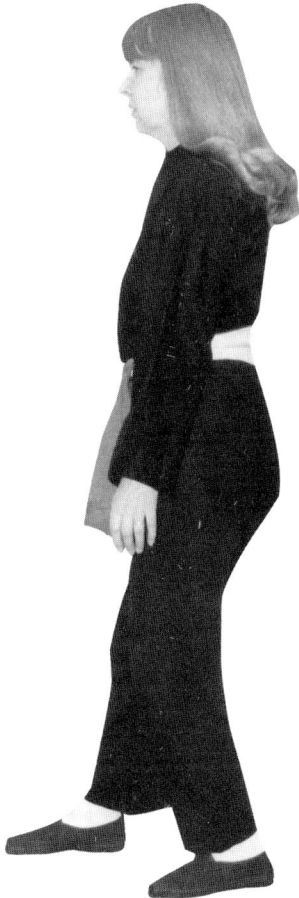

Eagle Stance

Eagle stance, place both heels together, toes pointing slightly outwards. Your weight should be evenly balanced between both legs.

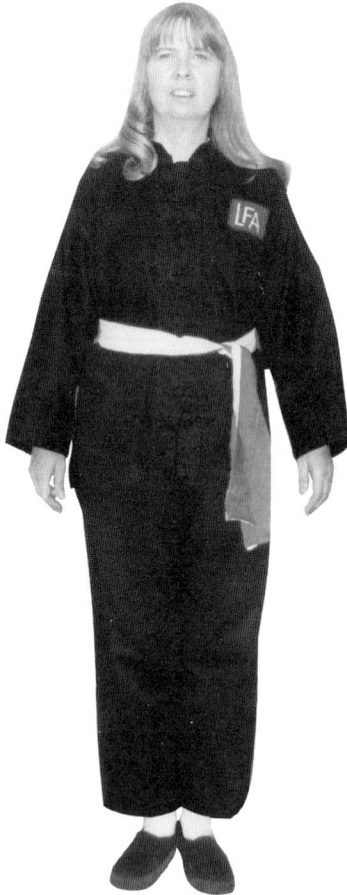

Extended Duck Stance

To achieve an Extended Left Duck Stance, step behind with your right foot so that it is slightly further across than you would normally step for a Duck Stance. Your weight is transferred onto your right leg with your right knee bent. Your left leg should be straight but not locked.

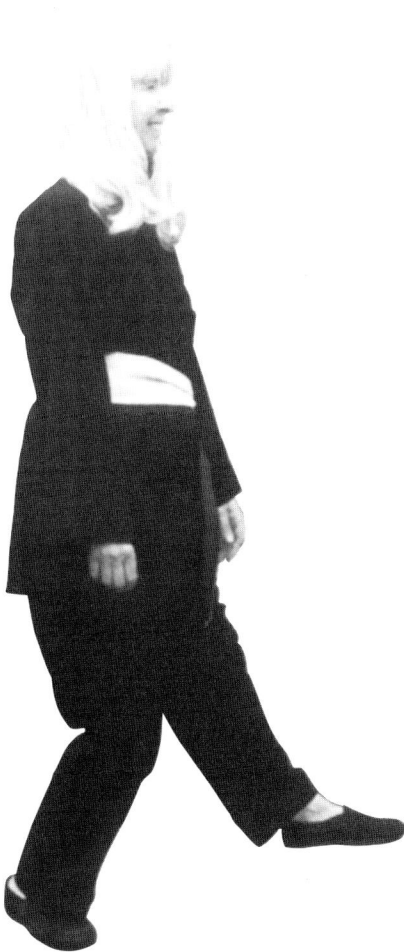

To achieve an Extended Right Duck Stance simply repeat the above on the opposite side.

Hawk Stance

To achieve a Right Hawk stance, move your weight onto your left leg (bending your knee slightly to aid your balance). Next move your right leg out directly behind you (bending your body forwards to create a natural line between your leg and your spine). Please remember there should be no strain, listen to your own body.

To achieve a Left Hawk stance, move your weight onto your right leg (bending your knee slightly to aid your balance). Next move your left leg out directly behind you.

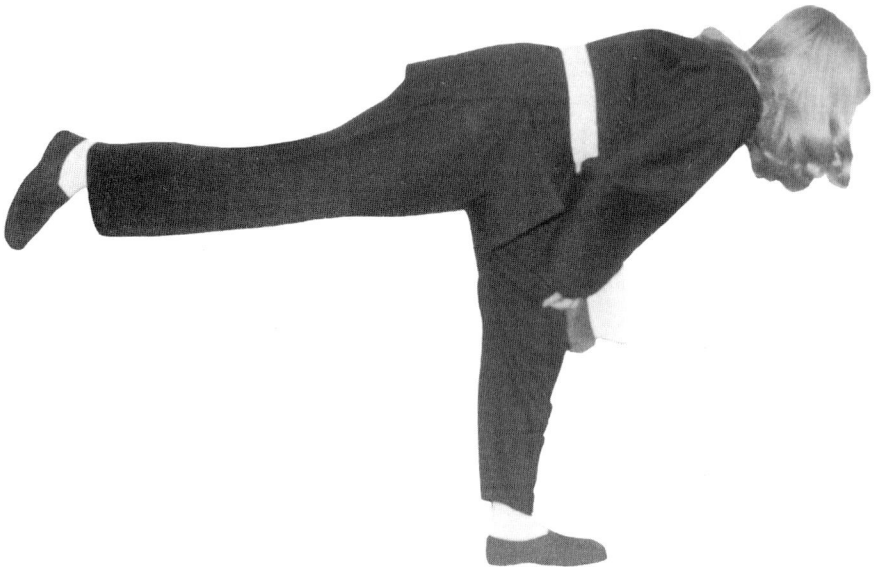

Leopard Stance

To achieve a Right Leopard stance take a pace off sideways to your right (bending your right knee and drifting your weight across). At the same time straighten your left leg.

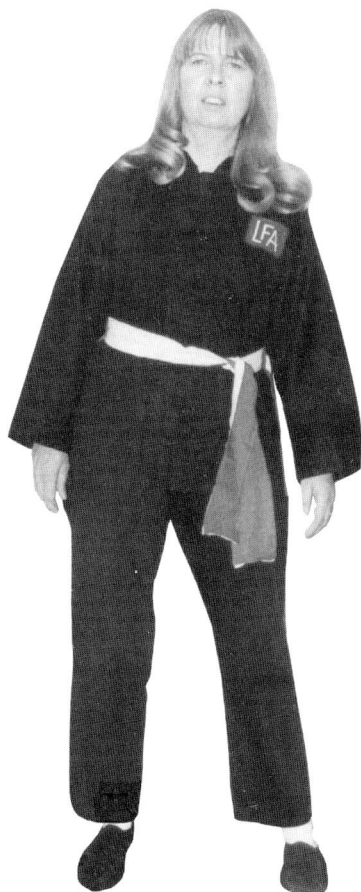

To achieve a Left Leopard stance take a pace off sideways to your left (bending your left knee and drifting your weight across). At the same time straighten your right leg.

Riding Horse Stance

To achieve a Riding Horse stance, stand with both feet slightly wider than shoulder width apart (both knees bent) your weight should be evenly distributed between both legs. Your body should be relaxed, without strain.

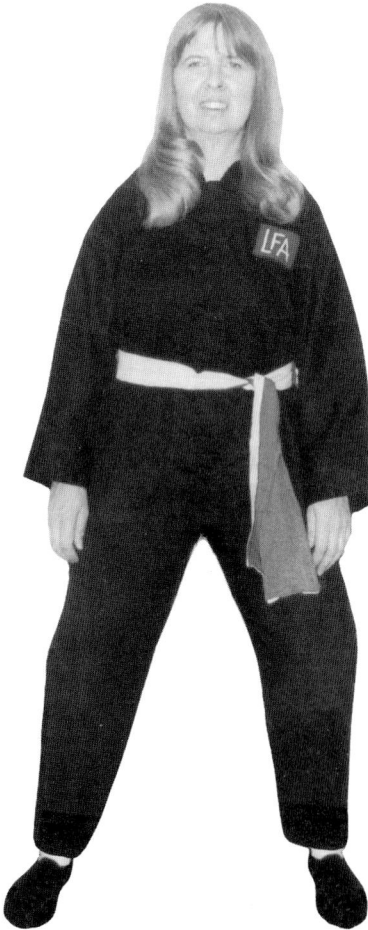

Scissors Stance

To achieve a Right Scissors stance drift your weight onto your left leg (bending your knee slightly). Now cross your right leg behind and slightly beyond your left leg, raising the heel of your right foot.

To achieve a Left Scissors stance drift your weight onto your right leg (bending your knee slightly). Now cross your left leg behind and slightly beyond your right leg, raising the heel of your left foot.

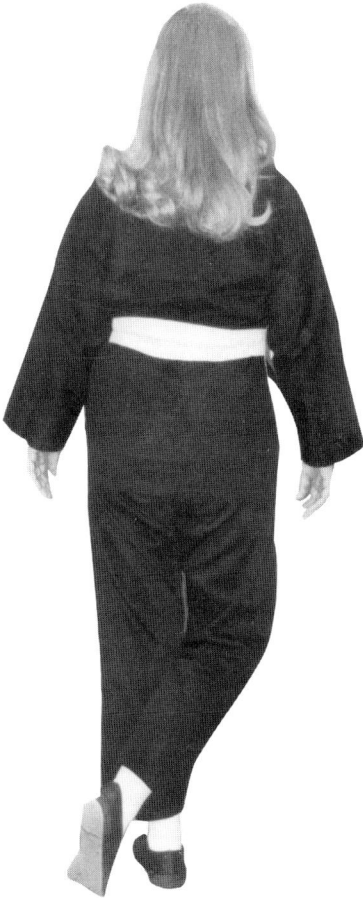

Snake Stance

To achieve a Right Snake stance take a small pace forwards with your right leg. Both knees are slightly bent, your weight is evenly distributed between both legs.
To achieve a Left Snake stance take a small pace forwards with your left leg. Both knees are slightly bent, your weight is evenly distributed between both legs.

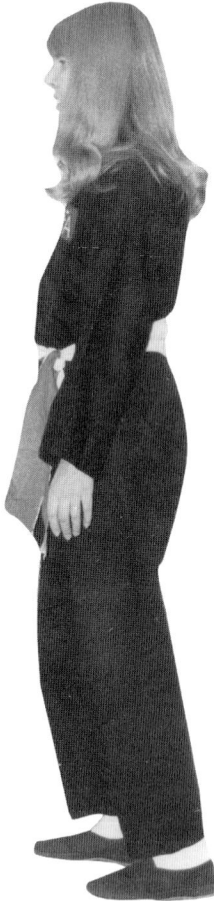

Stork Stance

To achieve a Right Stork stance move your weight onto your left leg (bending your left knee slightly to aid your balance). Now raise and bend your right leg moving your foot behind you.

To achieve a Left Stork stance move your weight onto your right leg (bending your right knee slightly to aid your balance). Now raise and bend your left leg moving your foot behind you.

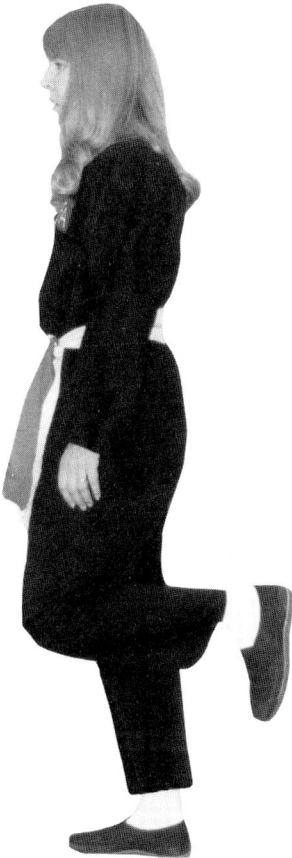

List of Stances 1 – 150

1	Eagle
2	Riding Horse
3	Right Dragon
4	Right Cat
5	Right Dragon
6	Right Dragon
7	Right Dragon
8	Left Dragon
9	Left Crane
10	Right Duck
11	Left Leopard
12	Right Leopard
13	Left Crane
14	Left Snake
15	Right Dragon
16	Right Duck
17	Riding Horse
18	Left Leopard
19	Right Crane
20	Right Dragon
21	Extended Left Duck
22	Left Stork
23	Right Scissors
24	Riding Horse

25	Left Crane
26	Right Crossed Legs
27	Left Crane
28	Left Dragon
29	Right Crane
30	Right Dragon
31	Left Duck
32	Left Cat
33	Right Crane
34	Right Dragon
35	Left Dragon
36	Right Dragon
37	Left Duck
38	Right Duck
39	Right Leopard
40	Right Leopard
41	Right Crossed Legs
42	Left Dragon
43	Left Duck
44	Right Dragon
45	Left Cat
46	Right Crossed Legs
47	Left Crane
48	Right Crane

49	Left Duck
50	Eagle
51	Left Dragon
52	Right Crane
53	Left Crane
54	Left Crane
55	Right Duck
56	Right Leopard
57	Right Scissors
58	Bear
59	Right Scissors
60	Bear
61	Right Dog
62	Right Crane
63	Left Dog
64	Left Crane
65	Right Scissors
66	Left Scissors
67	Left Leopard
68	Right Crane
69	Left Duck
70	Right Duck
71	Right Dragon
72	Left Dragon

73	Right Hawk
74	Left Duck
75	Right Duck
76	Right Leopard
77	Right Scissors
78	Right Dragon
79	Left Dragon
80	Right Leopard
81	Right Scissors
82	Right Stork
83	Right Dragon
84	Left Dragon
85	Right Duck
86	Left Dragon
87	Right Stork
88	Riding Horse
89	Right Crane
90	Left Crane
91	Left Dragon
92	Right Hawk
93	Right Dog
94	Right Dragon
95	Right Snake
96	Left Leopard

97	Right Crane
98	Right Scissors
99	Left Dragon
100	Left Crane
101	Right Scissors
102	Left Leopard
103	Right Crossed Legs
104	Left Dragon
105	Right Hawk
106	Right Dog
107	Right Dragon
108	Right Scissors
109	Left Dragon
110	Right Duck
111	Left Duck
112	Right Dragon
113	Left Scissors
114	Right Leopard
115	Left Stork
116	Left Crossed Legs
117	Right Dragon
118	Left Dragon
119	Right Dragon
120	Left Dragon

121	Right Dragon
122	Extended Left Duck
123	Right Crane
124	Right Dragon
125	Extended Left Duck
126	Right Crane
127	Left Scissors
128	Right Leopard
129	Left Scissors
130	Left Dragon
131	Right Dragon
132	Left Dragon
133	Left Duck
134	Right Cat
135	Left Crane
136	Right Chicken
137	Left Dragon
138	Bee
139	Right Leopard
140	Left Scissors
141	Right Dragon
142	Left Dog
143	Left Dragon
144	Right Duck

The LFA T'ai Chi Nunchaku Set
Movements 1 to 150

Starting Position

Stand in Eagle stance (both heels together, toes pointing slightly outwards) your weight is evenly distributed between both legs.

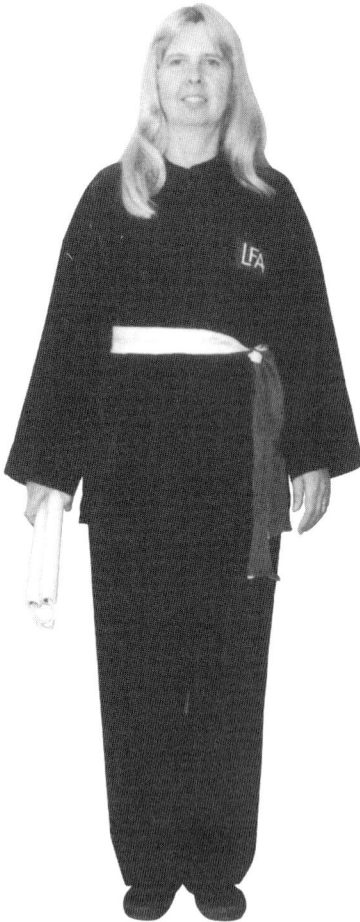

At the same time hold your nunchaku in your right hand, (side by side), thumb edge on the top. Your left arm hangs loosely by your left side.

Prepare

From Eagle stance take a pace off sideways with your left foot, into Bear stance (feet shoulder width apart); remember to place your left heel down first. Your nunchaku remain in your right hand,

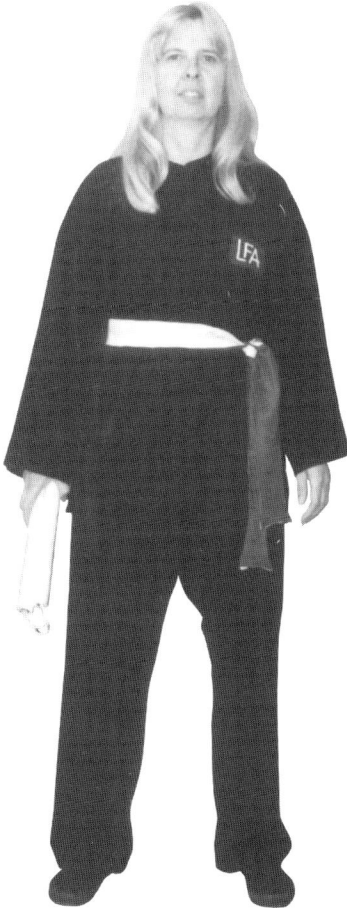

Number 1

From Bear stance draw your left foot to your right foot into Eagle stance (both heels together, toes pointing slightly outwards).

Your hands and nunchaku remain in the same position as they were in for 'Prepare'.

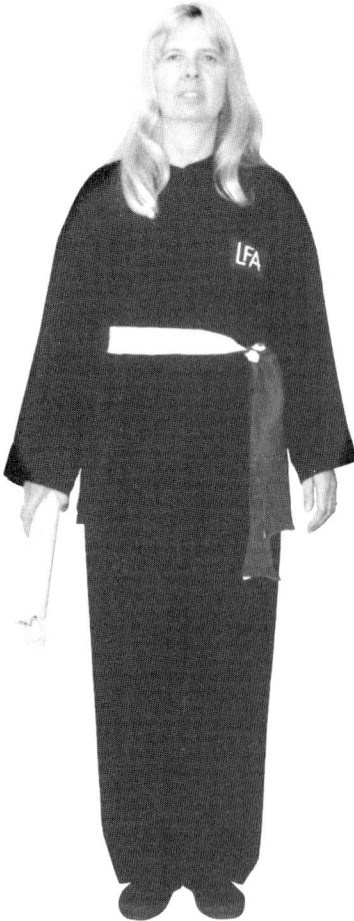

Number 2

From Eagle stance step out sideways with your left foot into Riding Horse stance (feet slightly wider than shoulder width apart, both knees bent).

At the same time let go of one part of your nunchaku. Holding the other part in your right hand, circle your right arm upwards swinging the free end of your nunchaku across to your left, catching it in your left hand (fingers curled over the top, thumb underneath). Both arms are now extended in front of your shoulders, elbows slightly bent outwards. (The nunchaku are horizontal with the cord pulled tight).

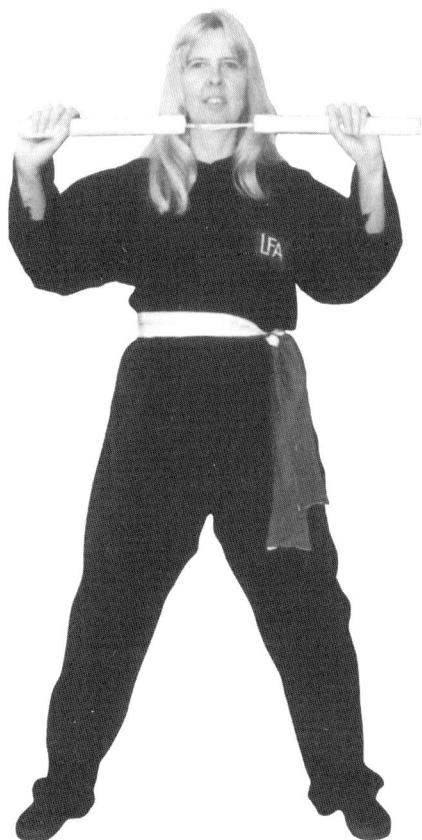

Number 3

From Riding Horse stance step forward with your right leg into Right Dragon stance. Remember to apply the principles of the Taoist Walk.

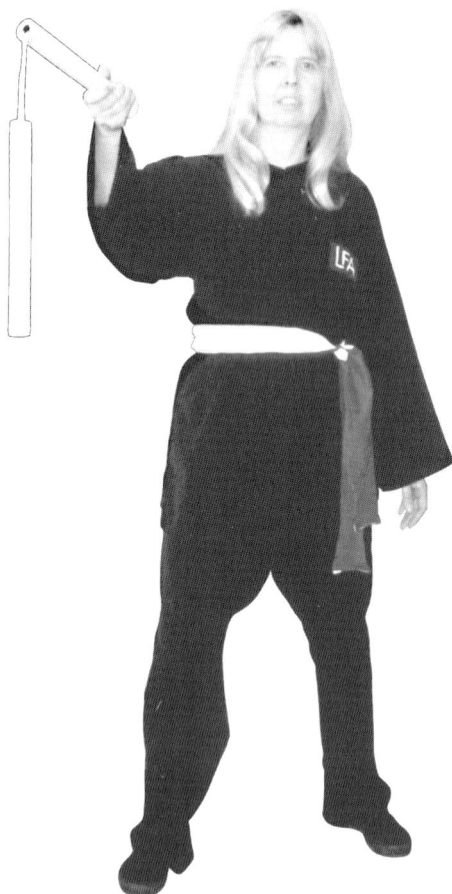

At the same time let go of your nunchaku with your left hand. With your right hand, swing the other part of your nunchaku forward by fully extending your right arm (your elbow is pointing down, your palm is facing up). This causes the free part of your nunchaku to circle up and over in front of the right side of your body.

Number 4

From Right Dragon stance slide your right foot back into Right Cat stance (left knee bent, the heel is raised on your right foot).

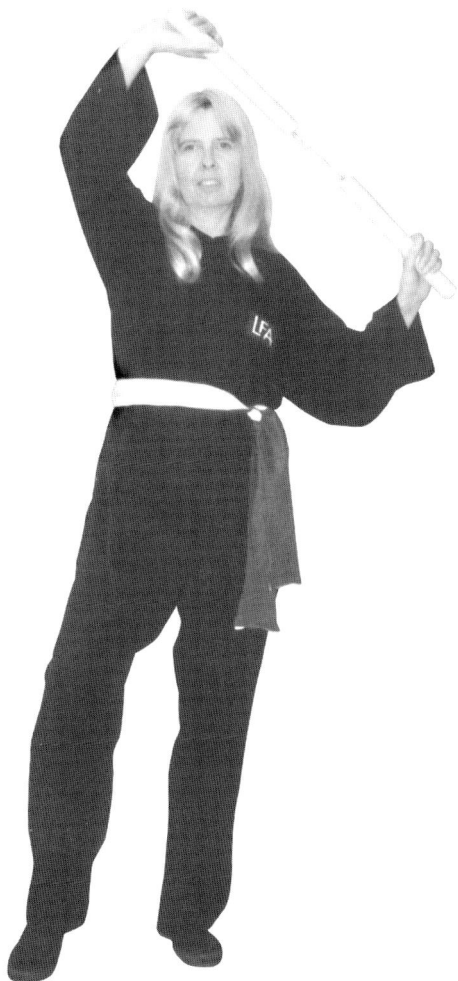

At the same time swing the free part of your nunchaku over to the left side of your body, catching it with your left hand. Your nunchaku are angled downwards to the left (the cord in the middle of your nunchaku is pulled tight).

Number 5

From Right Cat stance turn ninety degrees to your right into Right Dragon stance. Remember to apply the principles of the Taoist Walk. At the same time let go of your nunchaku with your left hand, swing the free part over the top as you make your turn to the right. Your right arm is extended forwards (your right thumb should now be on the top edge of your nunchaku).

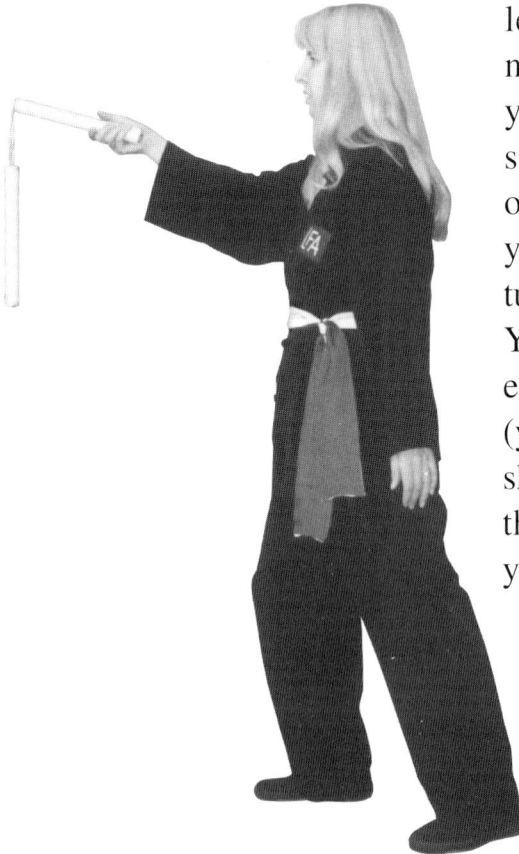

Number 6

Remain in Right Dragon stance for movement number six.

Still holding your nunchaku in your right hand, circle the free end downward towards the right hand side of your body and continue until your right hand is at the back of your waist (at your left side). Now exchange the nunchaku from your right hand to your left hand so that your left hand is now holding your nunchaku in front of you.

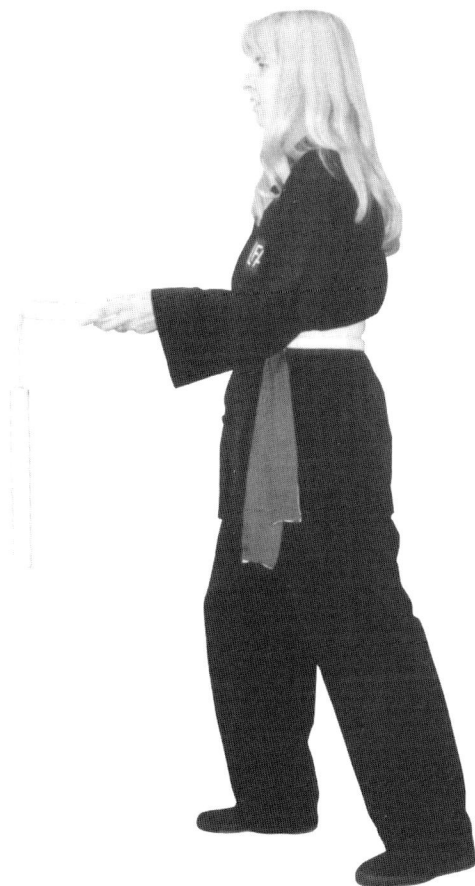

Number 7

Remain in Right Dragon stance for movement number seven.

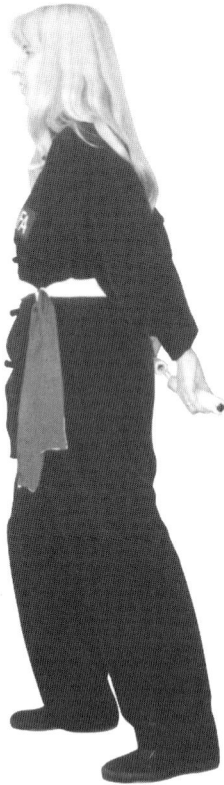

Circle your left hand (still holding your n u n c h a k u) round in front of your body. When it reaches your right side, exchange the nunchaku from your left hand to your right hand. Now swing the free end of your n u n c h a k u behind your back, catching it with your left hand.

Number 8

From Right Dragon stance turn one hundred and eighty degrees to your left into Left Dragon stance. Remember to apply the principles of the Taoist Walk. At the same time let go of your nunchaku with your right hand and swing them over the top as you make the turn with your body so that they finish extended forward (see photograph).

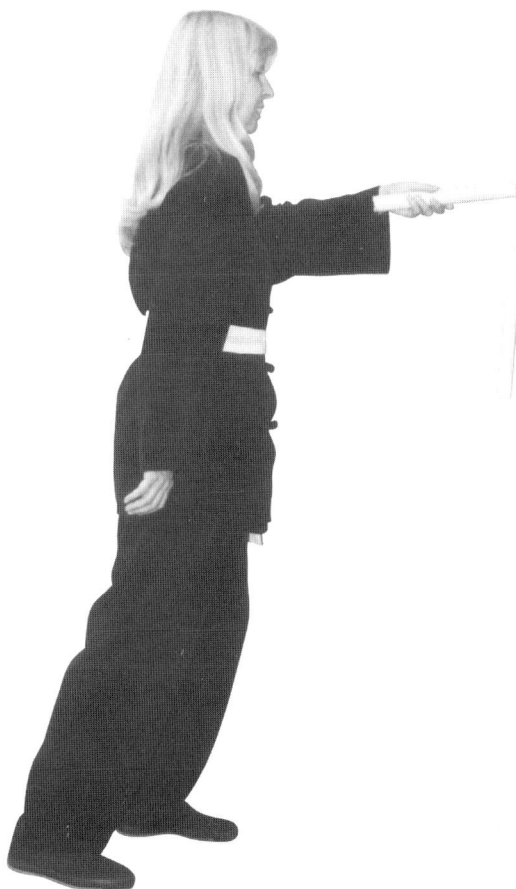

Number 9

From Left Dragon stance, raise your left leg into Left Crane stance (left knee bent, thigh parallel to the floor).

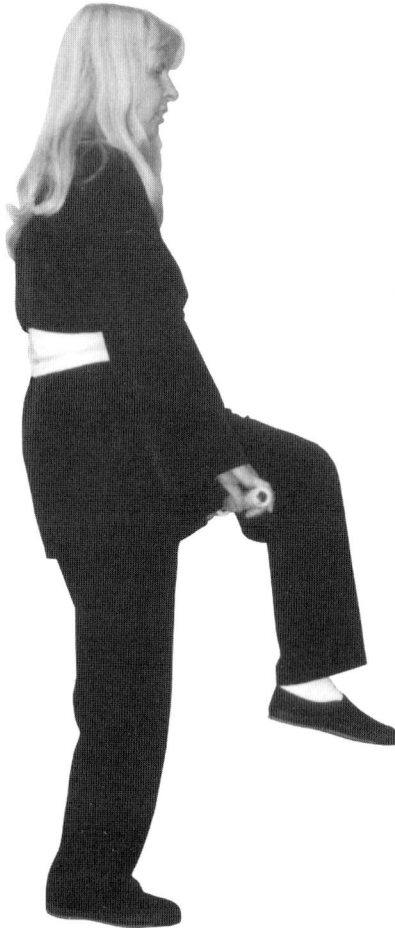

At the same time circle the free part of your nunchaku underneath your left leg, catching it with your right hand. Your nunchaku should now be horizontal (cord pulled tight).

Number 10

From Left Crane stance step behind with your left foot into Right Duck stance (remember to put your left heel down first).

At the same time let go of your nunchaku with your left hand, circle the free end up and over exchanging them from your right hand to your left hand. Continue to circle your nunchaku anticlockwise (behind your back), exchanging them from your left hand to your right hand (by your right hip). Now circle the free end of your nunchaku round and in front of your body, catching it with your left hand at shoulder height. Your nunchaku should be horizontal (cord pulled tight).

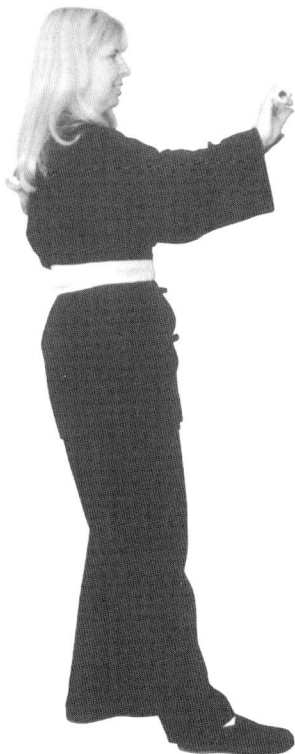

Number 11

From Right Duck stance turn ninety degrees to your right into Left Leopard stance (left leg bent, right leg straight).

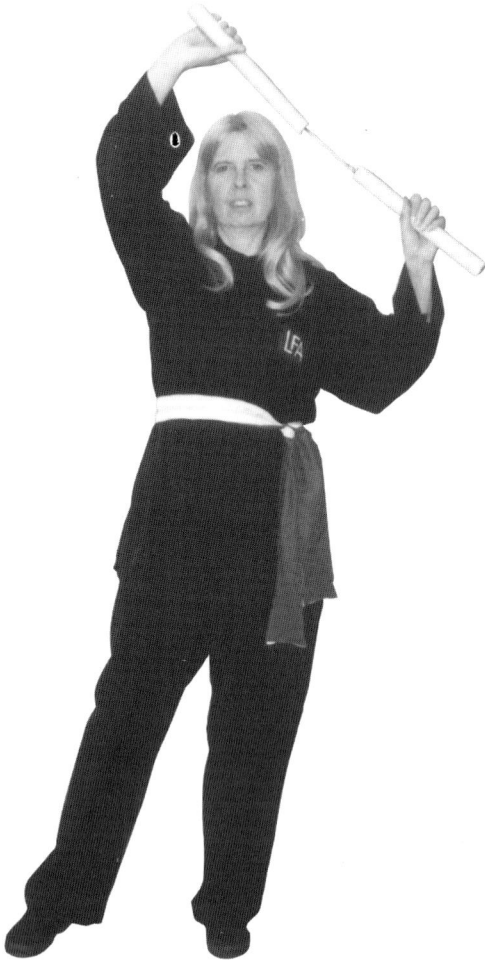

At the same time circle both arms over to the right then back to the left, to finish with your nunchaku angled downwards from right to left (see photograph).

Number 12

From Left Leopard stance transfer your weight across into Right Leopard stance (your feet do not move). Your right leg should now be bent and your left leg should be straight.

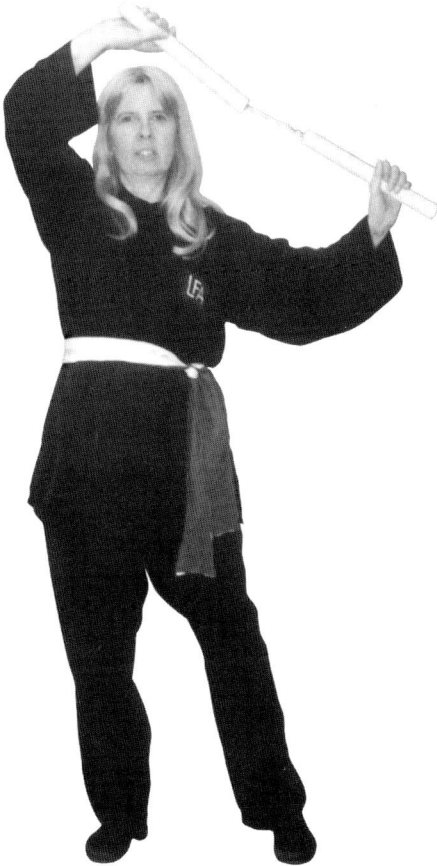

At the same time let go of your nunchaku with your left hand. Now circle your right hand out to your right (still in front of your body) catch the free end of your nunchaku with your left hand. Your hands and nunchaku should finish in the same position they were in for movement number eleven.

Number 13

From Right Leopard stance raise your left leg into Left Crane stance (left knee bent, thigh parallel to the floor).

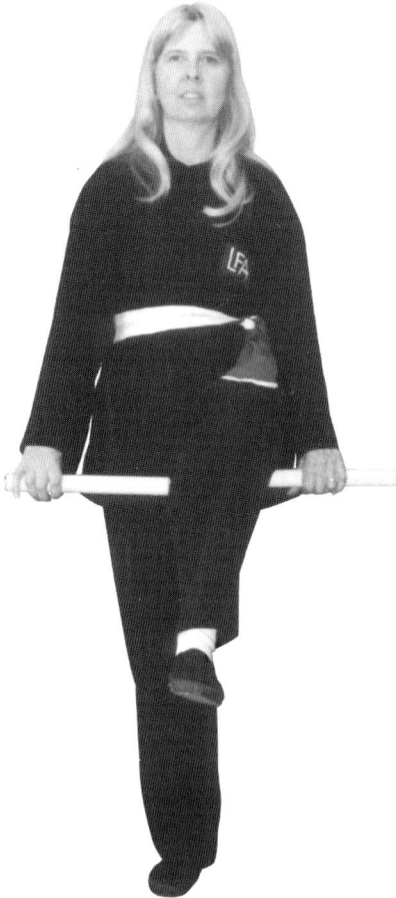

At the same time let go of your nunchaku with your left hand. Now circle them underneath your left leg catching the free end with your left hand. Your nunchaku should be horizontal, with the cord pulled tight.

Number 14

From Left Crane stance step forward into Left Snake stance (both knees bent, weight evenly distributed between both legs).

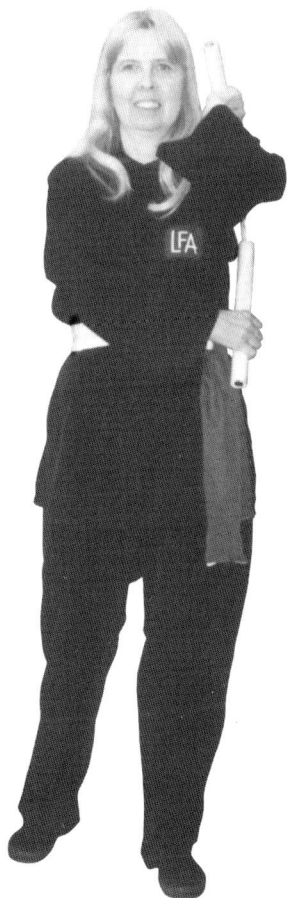

At the same time let go of your nunchaku with your right hand. Now swing the free end up and over your left shoulder. Catch the free end of your nunchaku with your right hand (your right arm is in front of your body, see photograph).

Number 15

From Left Snake stance step forward into Right Dragon stance. Remember to apply the principles of the Taoist Walk.

At the same time let go of your nunchaku with your left hand. Move your right hand forwards and upwards (right arm extended in front of your right shoulder with your right elbow bent outwards, knuckles facing you, thumb edge pointing down). Catch the free end of your nunchaku in your left hand. Your nunchaku are now vertical with the cord pulled tight. See photograph.

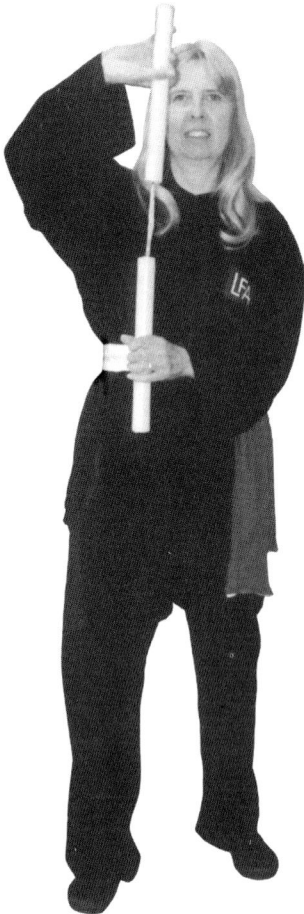

Number 16

From Right Dragon stance drift your weight back into Right Duck stance (right leg straight, left knee bent).

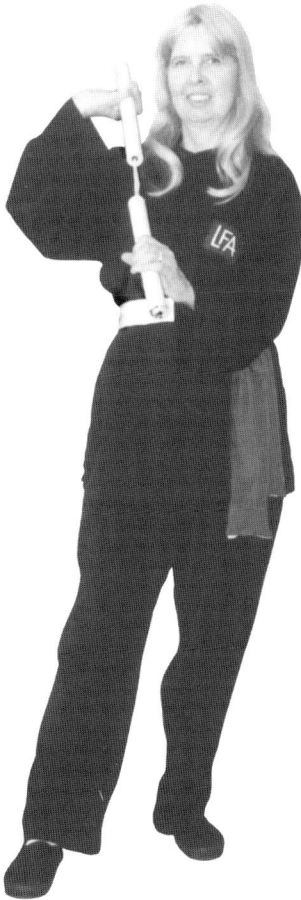

At the same time bend your right elbow more deeply, as your right hand moves back towards your right shoulder and your left hand moves slightly forwards. Your nunchaku should be angled downwards from your right shoulder.

Number 17

From Right Duck stance turn ninety degrees to your right into Riding Horse stance (feet slightly wider than shoulder width apart, both knees bent).

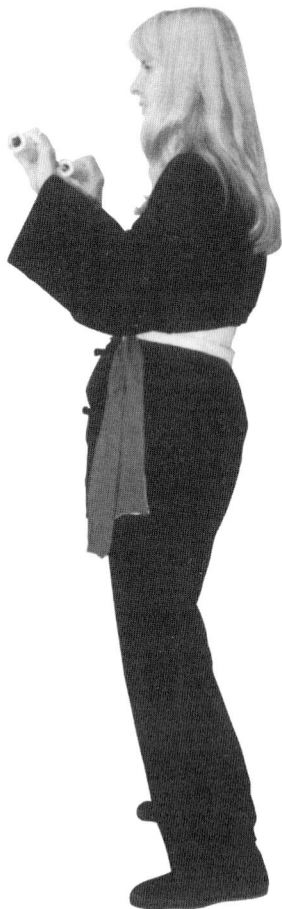

At the same time let go of your nunchaku with your left hand and swing the free end to your right (waist height). At the back of your waist, exchange them from your right hand to your left hand. Continue the circle, swinging your nunchaku to your left then up in front of your body. Catch the free end with your right hand, at shoulder height (cord pulled tight).

Number 18

From Riding Horse stance turn ninety degrees to your left into Left Leopard stance (left knee bent, right leg straight).

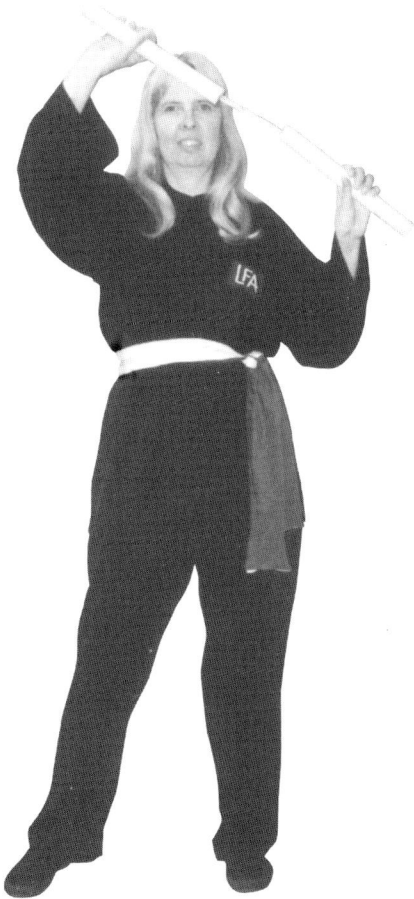

At the same time allow your nunchaku to move up and over, to finish angled down towards your left shoulder (see photograph).

Number 19

From Left Leopard stance turn two hundred and seventy degrees to your right into Right Crane stance (right knee bent, thigh parallel to the floor).

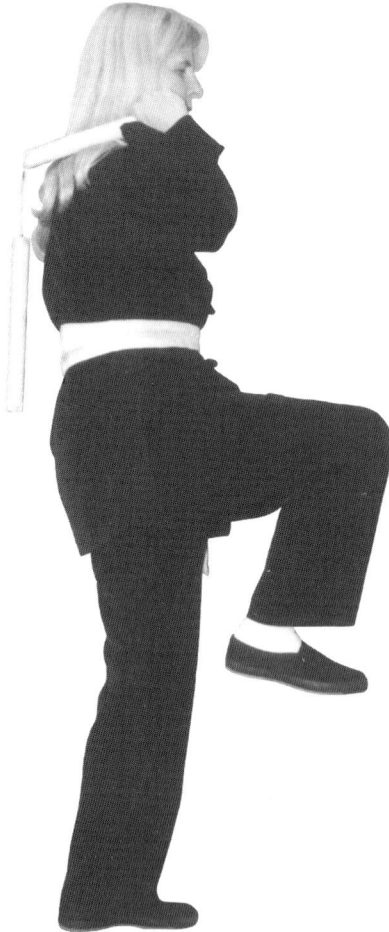

At the same time let go of your nunchaku with your left hand. Swing your nunchaku round as you make your turn, the cord is resting over your right shoulder. The free end is hanging over the back of your right shoulder. Your left hand is by your left side.

Number 20

From Right Crane stance step forward into Right Dragon stance. Remember to apply the principles of the Taoist Walk.

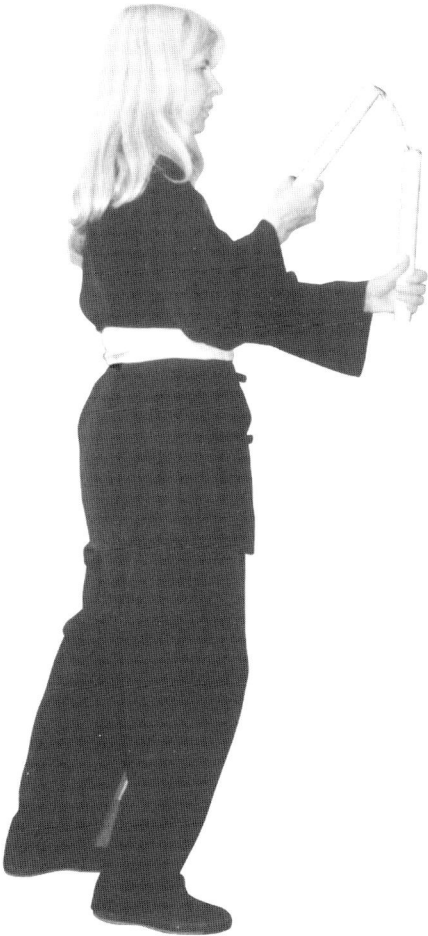

At the same time swing the free end of your nunchaku forwards and over, catching it with your left hand. The part of your nunchaku in your left hand is vertical. The part of your nunchaku in your right hand is angled in towards your body (see photograph).

Number 21

From Right Dragon stance step behind with your right foot into Extended Left Duck stance (this stance is wider and deeper than a normal Duck stance, please do not strain).

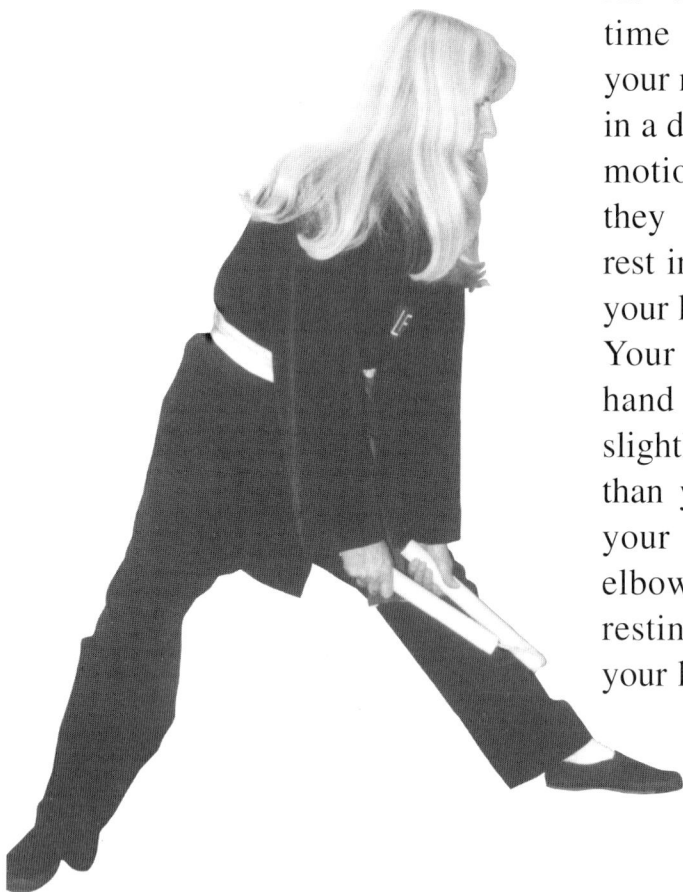

At the same time sweep your nunchaku in a downward motion, until they come to rest in front of your left thigh. Your right hand is slightly higher than your left, your left elbow is resting on your left hip.

Number 22

From Extended Left Duck stance turn ninety degrees to your left and step through into Left Stork stance. This is achieved by stepping through with your right foot first.

At the same time let go of your nunchaku with your right hand and swing them over your left shoulder. Catch the free end of your nunchaku behind your back with your right hand, (your nunchaku are angled downwards from left to right).

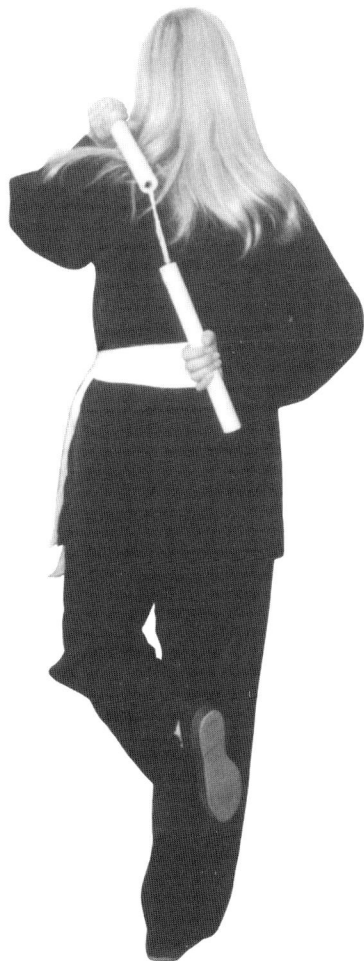

Number 23

From Left Stork stance cross your right leg behind your left leg into Right Scissors stance (both knees are slightly bent, your heel is raised on your right foot).

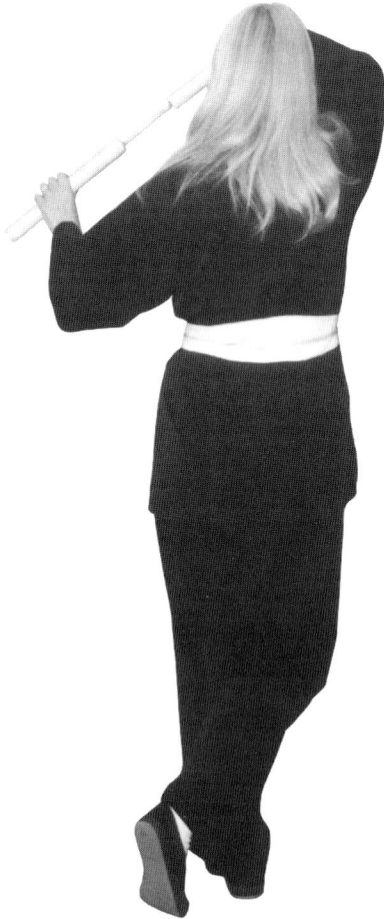

At the same time let go of your nunchaku with your left hand. With your right hand swing your nunchaku to the right so that they complete one full circle, then catch the free end with your left hand. Your nunchaku finish angled downwards from right to left.

Number 24

From Right Scissors stance turn one hundred and eighty degrees to your right into Riding Horse stance (you are once more facing the front). Both feet are slightly wider than shoulder width apart, both knees bent).

At the same time let go of your nunchaku with your left hand, circle the free end to the right and behind your back at waist height. Exchange your nunchaku from your right hand to your left hand. Continue to circle them round to the front of your body, swinging them upwards. Catch the free end of your nunchaku with your right hand, finishing with them at chest height. Both forearms are extended forwards with the elbows bent. The cord of your nunchaku should be tight with both ends angled downwards.

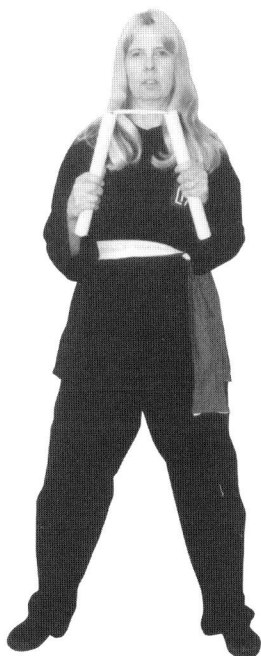

Number 25

From Riding Horse stance turn forty five degrees to your left into Left Crane stance (left knee bent, thigh parallel to the floor).

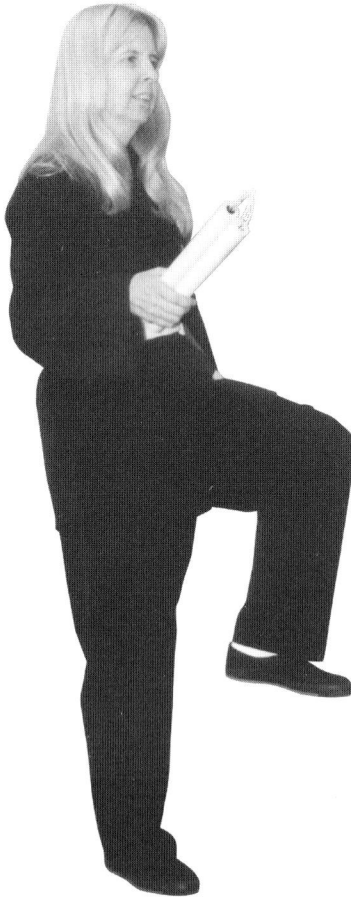

At the same time let go of your nunchaku with your left hand. Swing the free end forwards and over, catching it with your right hand (you are now holding both ends of your nunchaku in your right hand). Your right arm is bent with your elbow tucked into your waist.

Number 26

From Left Crane stance turn fortyfive degrees to your left into Right Crossed Legs stance. (your right leg is crossed in front of your left, your heel is raised on your right foot).

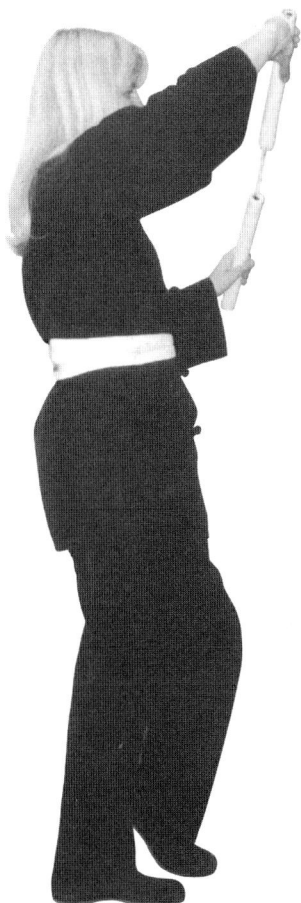

At the same time let go of <u>one end</u> of your nunchaku with your right hand and swing the free end round in one clockwise circle to the right before catching the free end with your left hand. Your nunchaku finishes angle downwards from right to left.

Number 27

From Right Crossed Legs stance place your right heel flat on the floor and raise your left leg into Left Crane stance (left knee bent, thigh parallel to the floor).

At the same time let go of your nunchaku with your left hand. With your right hand, swing the free end over your left shoulder, catching it behind your back with you left hand (see photograph).

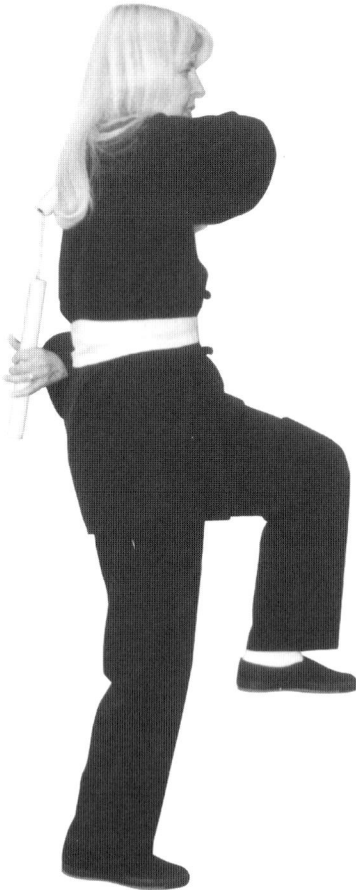

Number 28

From Left Crane stance step through into Left Dragon stance. Remember to apply the principles of the Taoist Walk.

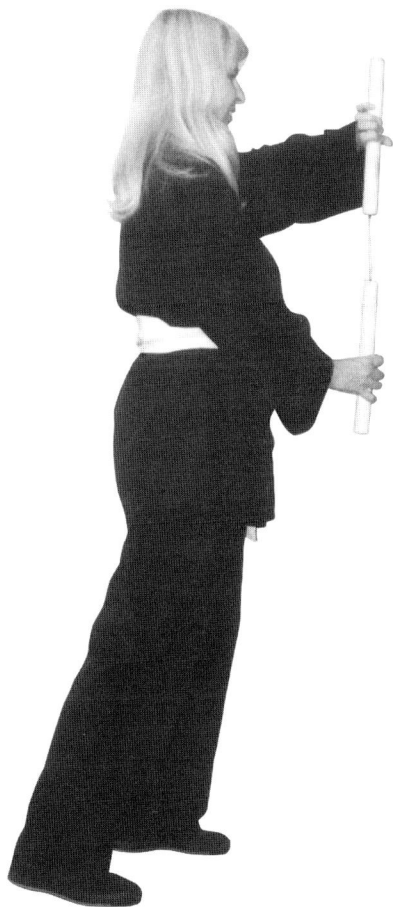

At the same time let go of your nunchaku with your right hand and pull the free end through with your left hand. Catch the free end with your right hand. Your n u n c h a k u should finish vertical in front of the left side of your body.

Number 29

From Left Dragon stance raise your right leg into Right Crane stance (right knee bent, thigh parallel to the floor).

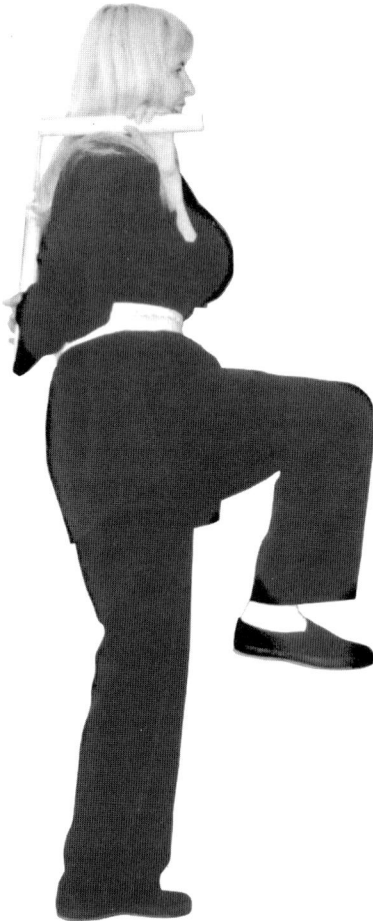

At the same time let go of your nunchaku with your right hand and swing the free end over your right shoulder, catching it with your right hand. The other end of your nunchaku should finish in a straight line behind your right shoulder

Number 30

From Right Crane stance step forwards into Right Dragon stance. Remember to apply the principles of the Taoist Walk.

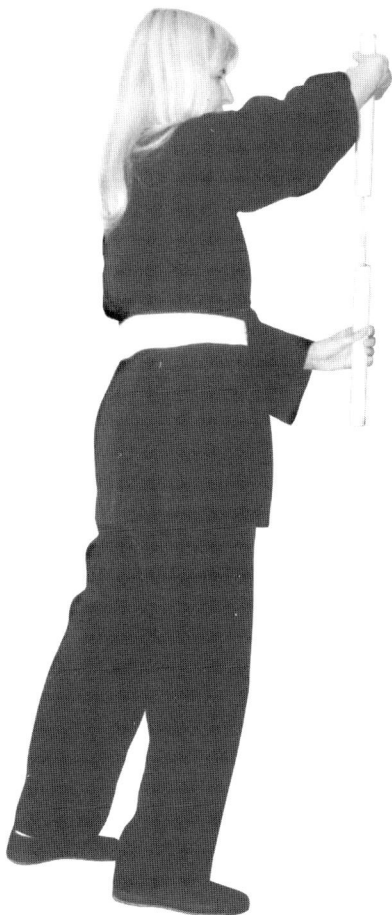

At the same time let go of your nunchaku with your left hand and pull the free end through with your right hand. Catch the free end of your nunchaku with your left hand, finishing with your nunchaku vertical in front of the right side of your body.

Number 31

From Right Dragon stance turn one hundred and eighty degrees to the left into Left Duck stance (right leg bent, left leg straight).

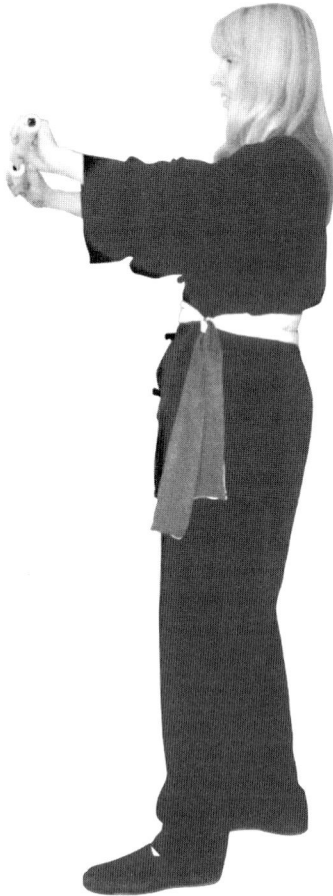

At the same time let go of your nunchaku with your left hand and allow the free end to swing round with the movement of your body. Catch the free end with your left hand. Your nunchaku finish horizontal at shoulder height.

Number 32

From Left Duck stance draw your left foot back into Left Cat stance (right knee bent, the heel of your left foot is raised).

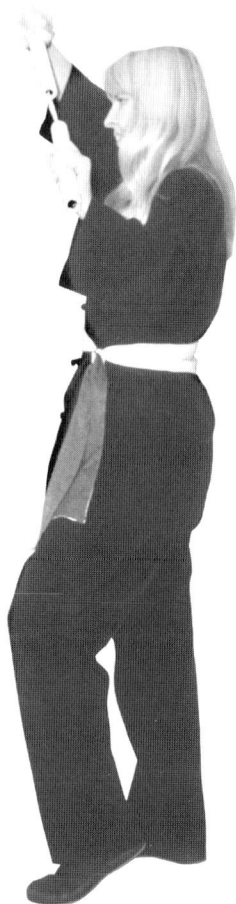

At the same time let go of your nunchaku with your left hand. With your right hand, swing the free end of your nunchaku to your right, completing a full clockwise circle. Catch the free end with your left hand (finishing with your nunchaku angled down from right to left). See photograph.

Number 33

From Left Cat stance place the heel of your left foot flat on the floor turning it fortyfive degrees to the left. Now raise your right leg into Right Crane stance (right knee bent, thigh parallel to the floor).

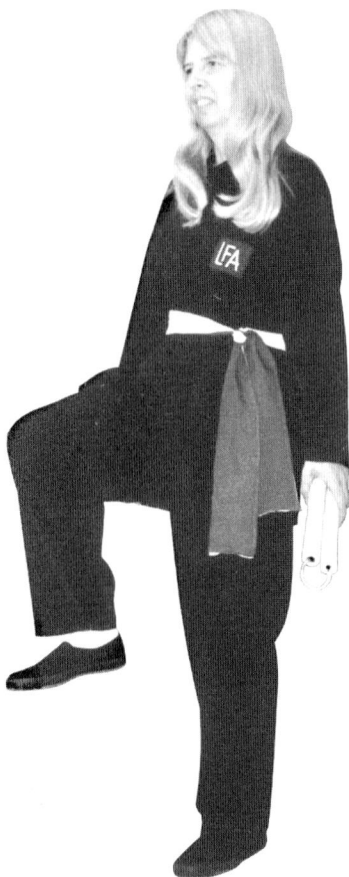

At the same time let go of your nunchaku with your right hand. Swing the free end forwards and over, catching it with your left hand, (so that you are now holding both ends of your nunchaku in your left hand). Your left elbow is tucked into the left side of your waist.

Number 34

From Right Crane stance step forty five degrees to the right into Right Dragon stance. Remember to apply the principles of the Taoist Walk.

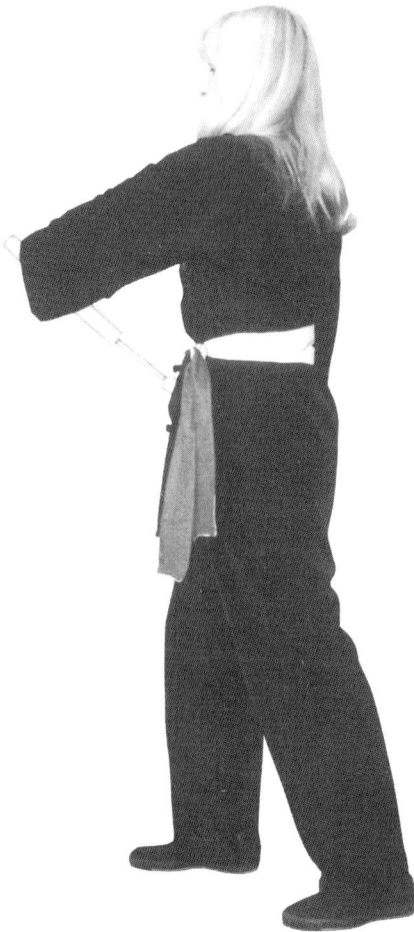

At the same time let go of <u>one end</u> of your nunchaku and swing it over to the right side of your body, catching it with your right hand. Your nunchaku are angled upwards from your right hip.

Number 35

From Right Dragon stance step forwards into Left Dragon stance. Remember to apply the principles of the Taoist Walk.

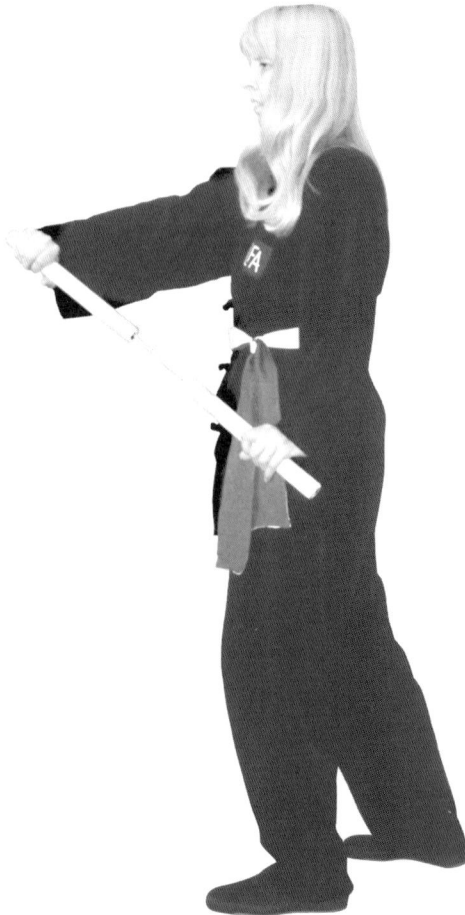

At the same time let go of your nunchaku with your left hand and swing the free end over to the left side of your body catching it with your left hand. Your nunchaku finish angled upwards from your left hip.

Number 36

From Left Dragon stance step forward into Right Dragon stance. Remember to apply the principles of the Taoist Walk.

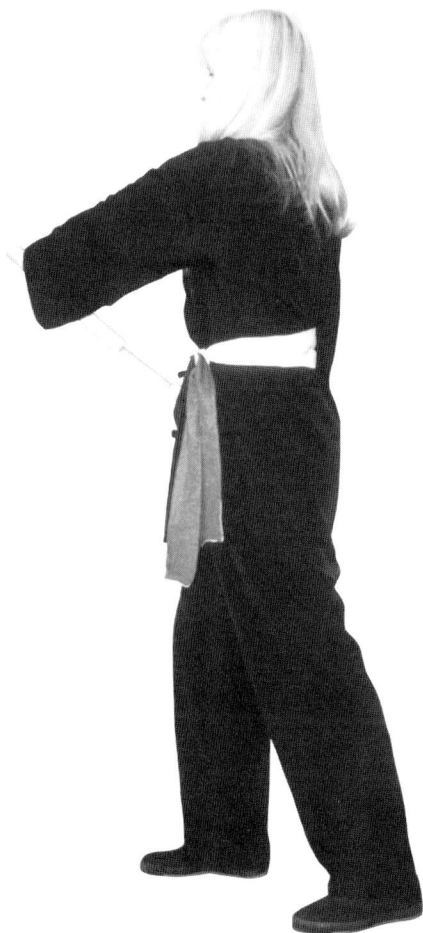

At the same time let go of your nunchaku with your right hand and swing the free end over to the right side of your body, catching it with your right hand. Your nunchaku finish angled upwards from your right hip.

Number 37

From Right Dragon stance step behind with your right foot into Left Duck stance (right knee bent, left leg straight.

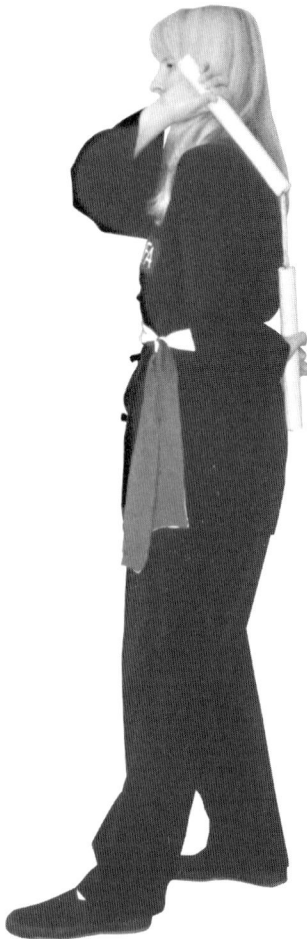

At the same time let go of your nunchaku with your left hand, swing the free end over your left shoulder, catching it behind your back with your left hand.

Number 38

From Left Duck stance step behind with your left foot into Right Duck stance (left knee bent, right leg straight).

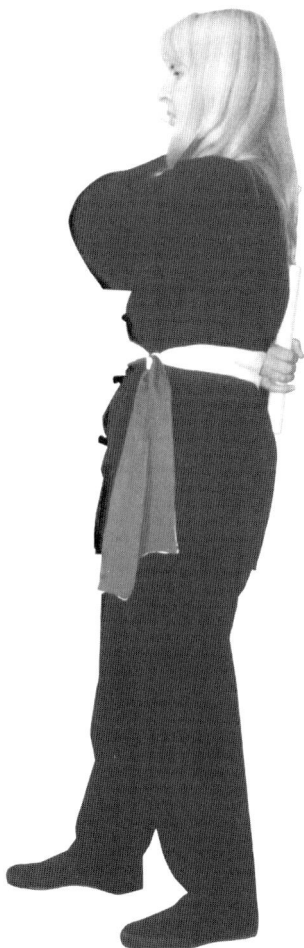

At the same time let go of your nunchaku with your right hand. Pull the free end through, then over your right shoulder, catching it behind your back with your right hand.

Number 39

From Right Duck stance turn ninety degrees to your left into Right Leopard stance (right knee bent, left leg straight).

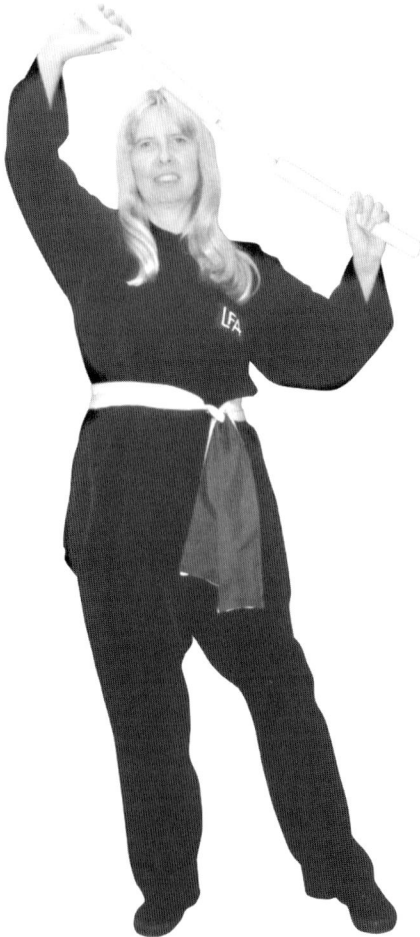

At the same time let go of your nunchaku with your left hand. Using your right hand, pull the free end of your nunchaku through and circle your right arm to the right (making one complete circle), before catching your nunchaku in your left hand. Your nunchaku are angled downwards from right to left.

Number 40

From Right Leopard stance turn one hundred and eighty degrees to your right into Right Leopard stance. At the same time let go of your nunchaku with your right hand. The free end of your nunchaku, swings round as you make your turn. Catch the free end with your right hand. Your nunchaku finish horizontal at shoulder height .

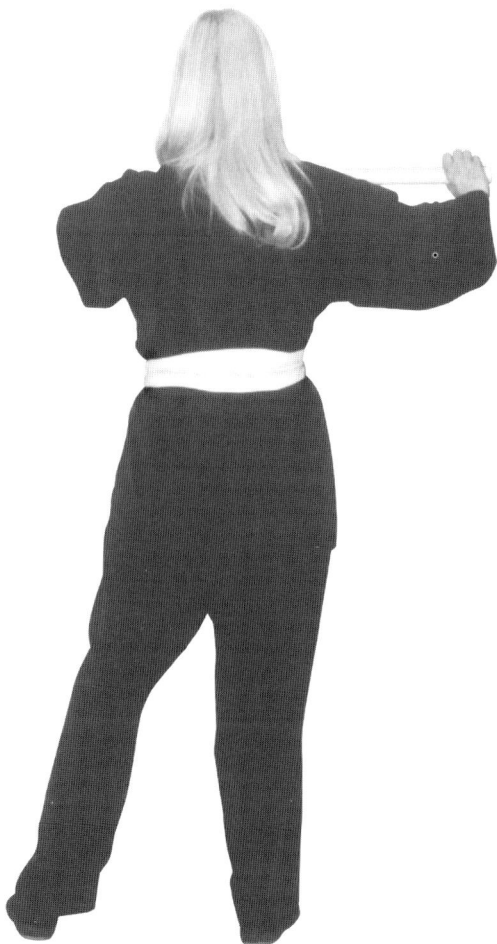

Number 41

From Right Leopard stance cross your right foot in front of your left leg into Right Crossed Legs stance (both knees bent, the heel is raised on your right foot).

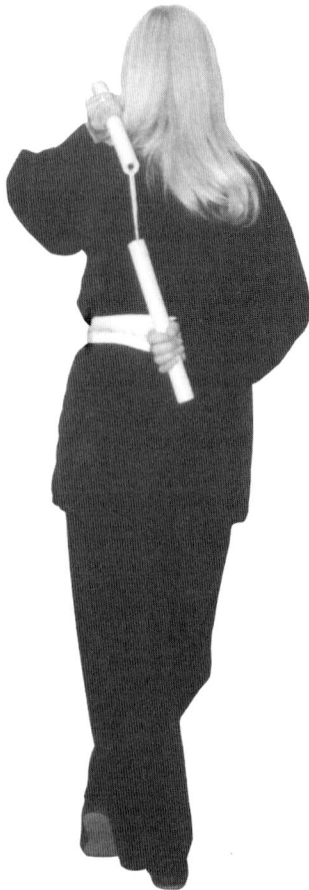

At the same time let go of your nunchaku with your right hand. Swing the free end over your left shoulder, catching it with your right hand behind your back at your left side. Your nunchaku finish on the diagonal (left hand high – right hand low).

Number 42

From Right Crossed Legs stance step forwards into Left Dragon stance. Remember to apply the principles of the Taoist Walk.

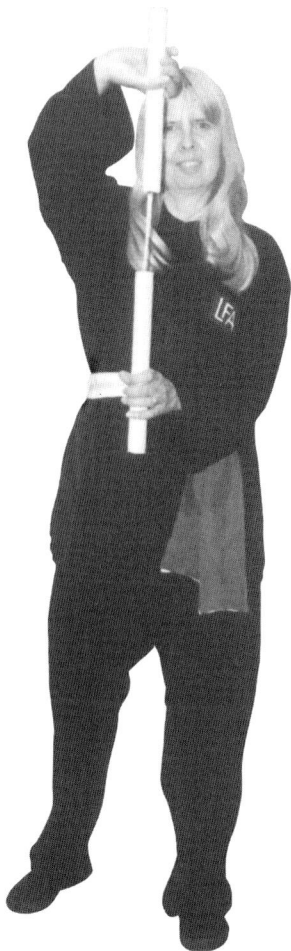

At the same time let go of your nunchaku with your left hand and pull the free end through, catching it with your left hand. Your nunchaku finish vertical (right hand high – left hand low). Note: the p h o t o g r a p h shows the front view, but the actual stance is with the back facing the camera.

Number 43

From Left Dragon stance transfer your weight back into Left Duck stance (right leg bent, left leg straight). At the same time (keeping hold of both ends of your nunchaku), allow your right arm to bend in towards your body (bending at the elbow), while your left hand moves upwards. Note: the photograph shows the front view, but the actual stance is with the back facing the camera.

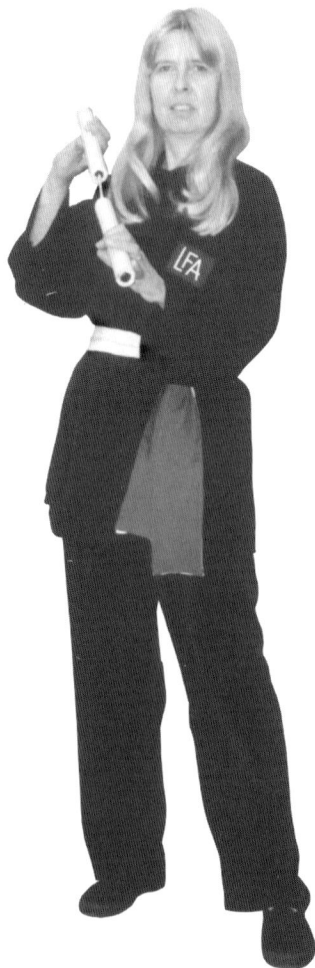

Number 44

From Left Duck stance turn one hundred and eighty degrees to your right into Right Dragon stance.

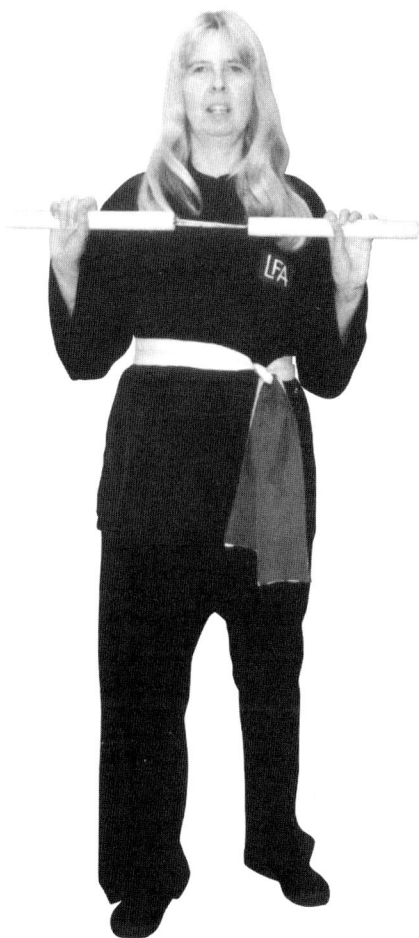

At the same time let go of your nunchaku with your left hand and allow the free end to swing to your right. Now circle your nunchaku behind your back exchanging them from your right hand to your left hand. Continue the circle catching the free end in your right hand. Your nunchaku finish horizontal at chest height.

Number 45

From Right Dragon step through into Left Cat stance (right knee bent, the heel is raised on your left foot). At the same time let go of your nunchaku with your right hand and swing the free end over your left shoulder catching it with your right hand behind your back. Your nunchaku are angled downwards from left to right.

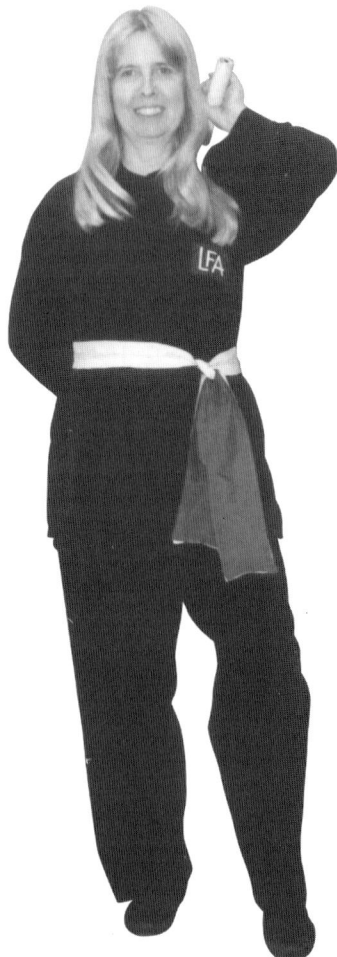

Number 46

From Left Cat stance place your left heel flat on the floor and cross your right foot in front of your left leg into Right Crossed Legs stance.

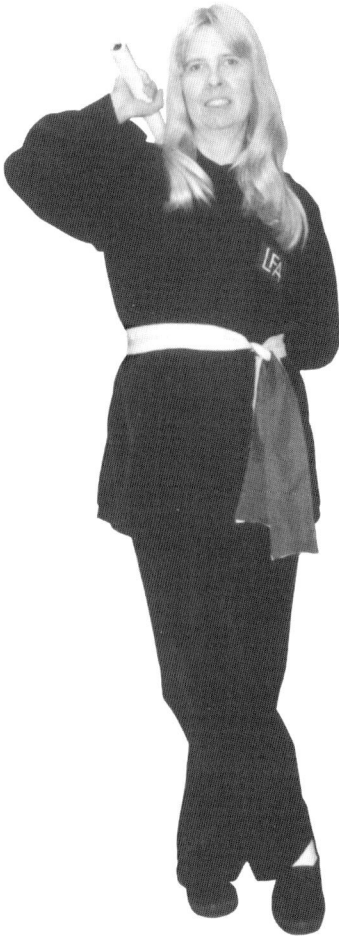

At the same time let go of your nunchaku with your left hand and pull the free end through with your right hand, then over your right shoulder. Catch the free end of your nunchaku with your left hand behind your back.

Your nunchaku finish angled downwards from right to left.

Number 47

From Right Crossed Legs stance place your right heel flat on the floor and raise your left leg into Left Crane stance (left knee bent, thigh parallel to the floor).

At the same time let go of your nunchaku with your right hand, swing the free end out to the left then over so that it is above your left thigh. Now exchange your nunchaku from your left hand to your right hand, swing the free end underneath your left leg catching it with your left hand.

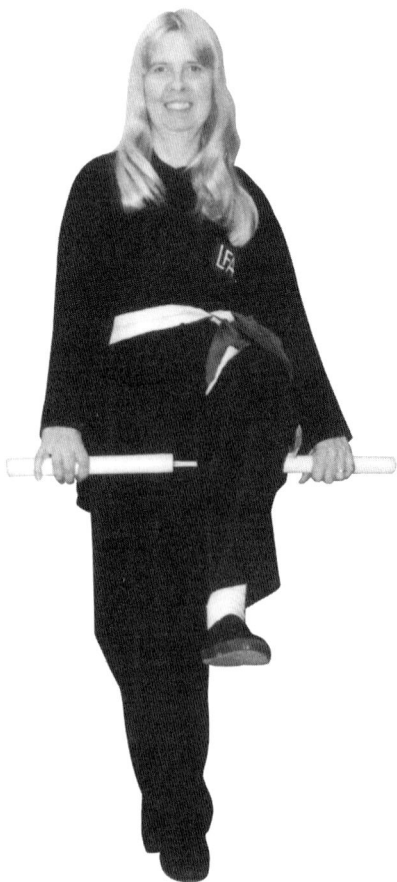

Number 48

From Left Crane stance place your left foot flat on the floor and raise your right leg into Right Crane stance (right knee bent, thigh parallel to the floor).

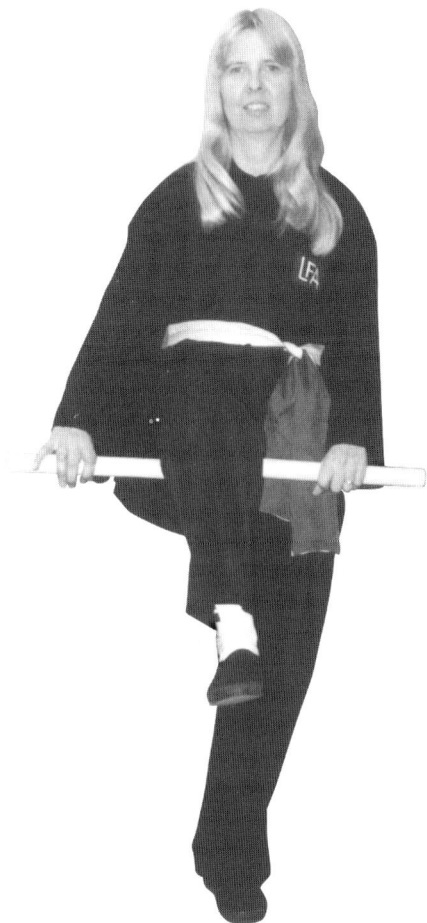

At the same time let go of your nunchaku with your right hand, swing the free end out to the left, then over and above your right thigh. Exchange your nunchaku from your left hand to your right hand, now swing the free end underneath your right leg, catching it with your left hand.

Number 49

From Right Crane stance, step behind with your right foot into Left Duck stance (right knee bent, left leg straight).

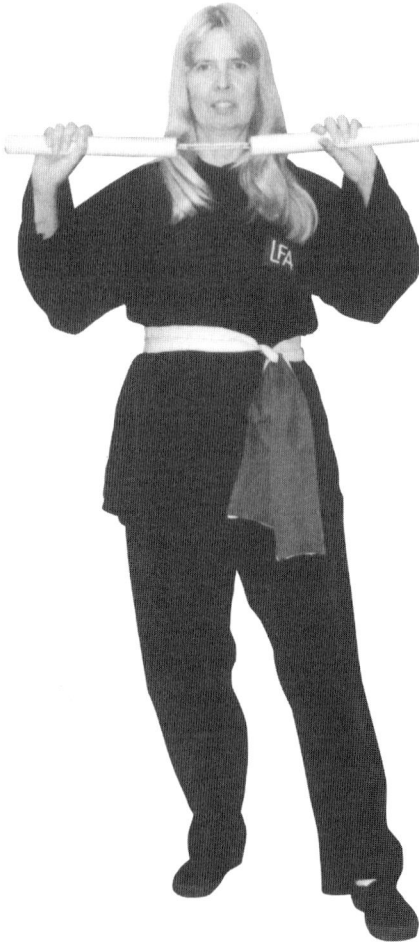

At the same time let go of your nunchaku with your right hand, exchange them from your left hand to your right hand as you circle your nunchaku in front of you and then round behind your back. Exchange them from your right hand to your left hand (continue the circle round) catching the free end with your right hand, at shoulder height.

Number 50

From Left Duck stance step forward with your right foot into Eagle stance (both heels together, toes pointing slightly outwards).

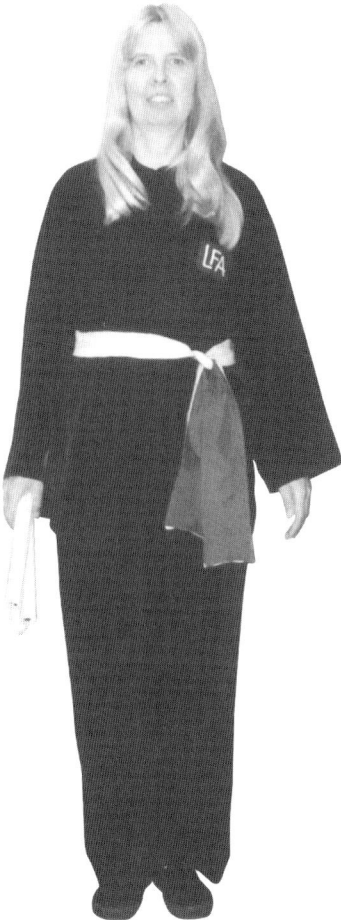

At the same time place both ends of the nunchaku together in your right hand. Both hands finish by your sides.

Number 51

From Eagle stance turn ninety degrees to the left into Left Dragon stance. Remember to apply the principles of the Taoist Walk.

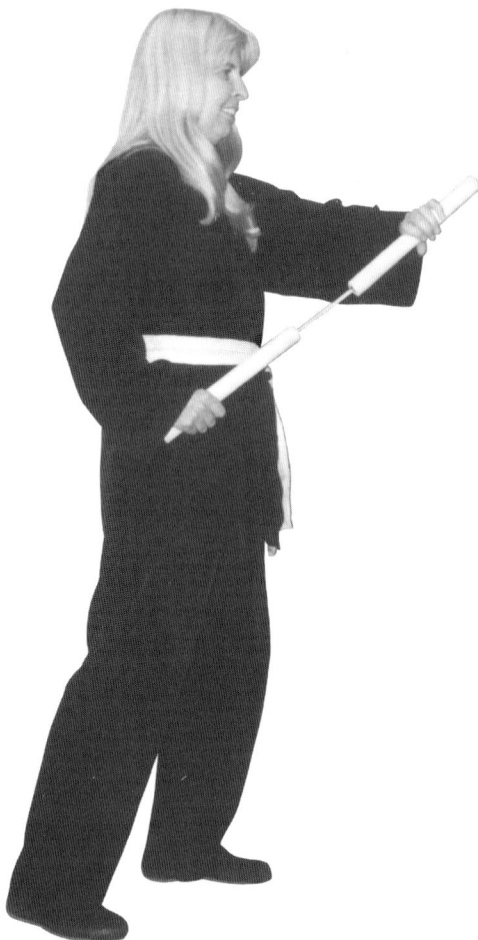

At the same time release one end of your nunchaku and circle your right arm over (behind you) then forwards, catching your nunchaku with your left hand. Your nunchaku finish angled upwards from your right hip.

Number 52

From Left Dragon stance raise your right leg into Right Crane stance (right knee bent, thigh parallel to the floor).

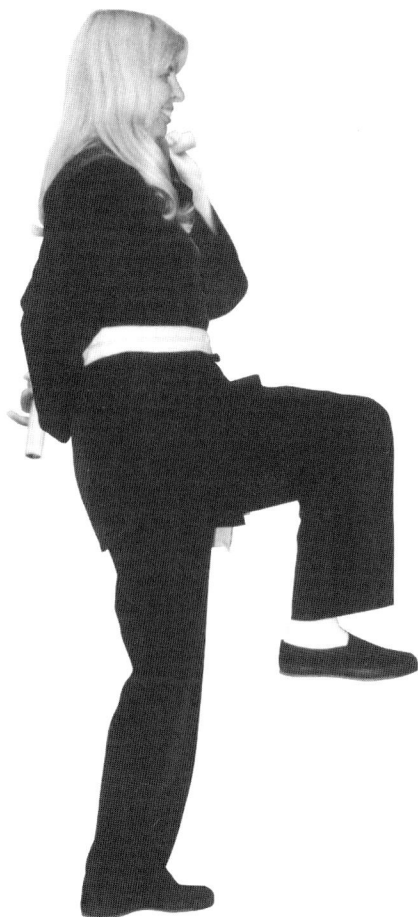

At the same time left go of your nunchaku with your right hand and swing the free end over your left shoulder, catching it behind your back with your right hand.

Number 53

From Right Crane stance lower your right foot and raise your left leg into Left Crane stance (left knee bent, thigh parallel to the floor).

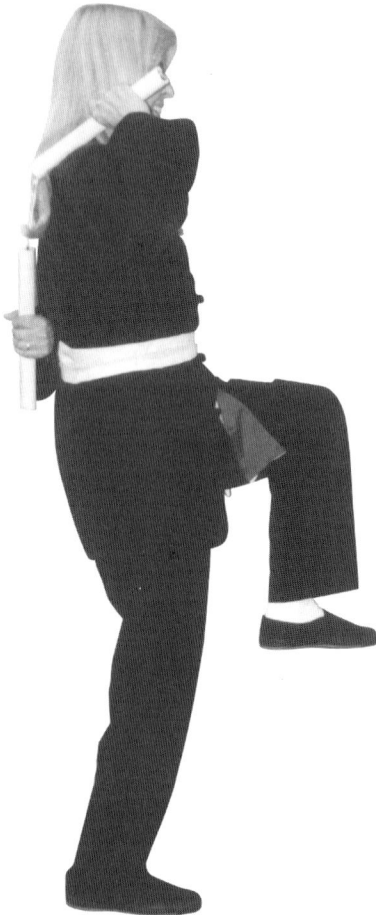

At the same time left go of your nunchaku with your left hand and pull the free end through and then over your right shoulder, catching the free end behind your back with your left hand.

Number 54

Stay in Left Crane stance for movement number fiftyfour.

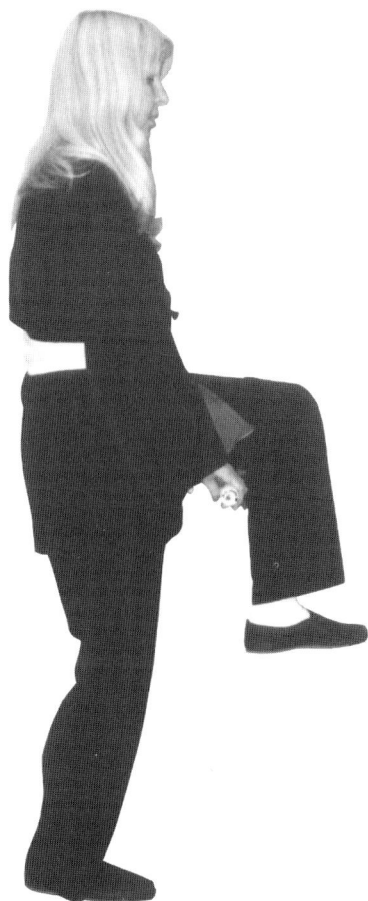

Let go of your nunchaku with your right hand and pull the free end round and through, now exchange your nunchaku from your left hand to your right hand. Swing the free end underneath your left leg, catching it with your left hand.

Number 55

From Left Crane stance step behind with your left foot into Right Duck stance (left knee bent, right leg straight).

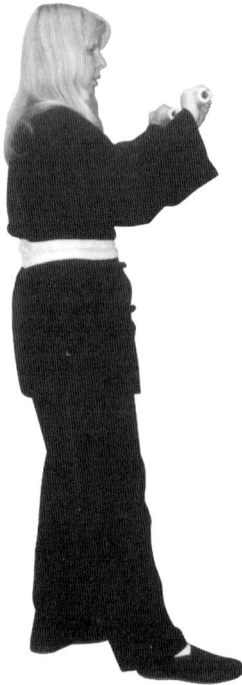

At the same time let go of your nunchaku with your right hand. Circle your left hand over to the right transferring your nunchaku from your left hand for your right hand. Circle your right hand behind your back exchanging your nunchaku from your right hand to your left hand then catch the free end in front of your body with your right hand.

Number 56

From Right Duck stance turn ninety degrees to the left into Right Leopard stance (right knee bent, left leg straight).

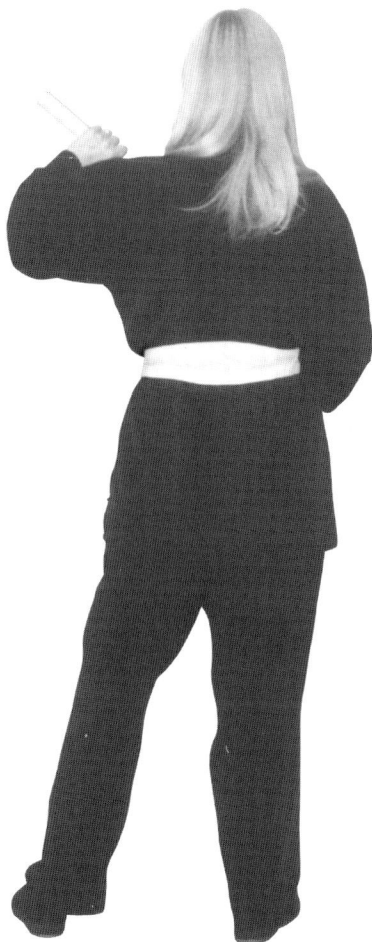

At the same time let go of your nunchaku with your left hand and complete one clockwise circle with the free end of your nunchaku before catching it with your left hand. Your nunchaku are angled downwards from left to right.

Number 57

From Right Leopard stance cross your right foot behind your left leg into Right Scissors stance (both knees are bent, the heel is raised on your right foot).

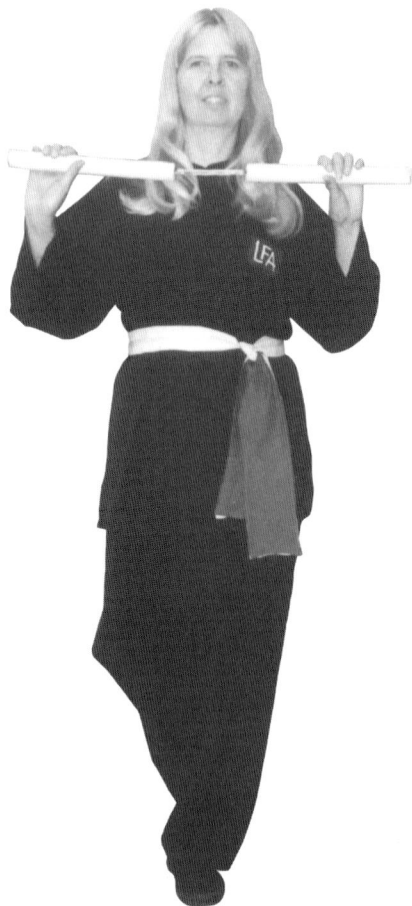

At the same time let go of your nunchaku with your left hand and circle your right hand behind your back transferring your nunchaku from your right hand to your left hand. Now continue the circle with your left hand swinging the free end of your nunchaku round so that you can catch it with your right hand. Your nunchaku finish horizontal at shoulder height.

Note: the photograph shows the front view, but the actual stance is with the back facing the camera.

Number 58

From Right Scissors stance place your right heel flat on the floor and step sideways with your left foot into Bear stance (feet shoulder width apart).

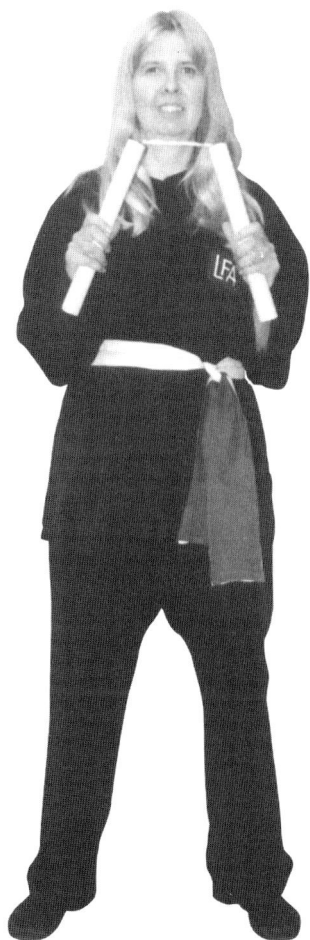

At the same time let go of your nunchaku with your left hand, circle your right hand behind your back, transferring your nunchaku from your right hand to your left hand. Now complete the circle with your left hand swinging the free end round, to be caught by your right hand. The cord is pulled tight, both ends are pointing downwards and slightly inwards towards the body.

Note: the photograph shows the front view, but the actual stance is with the back facing the camera.

Number 59

From Bear stance cross your right foot behind your left leg into Right Scissors stance.

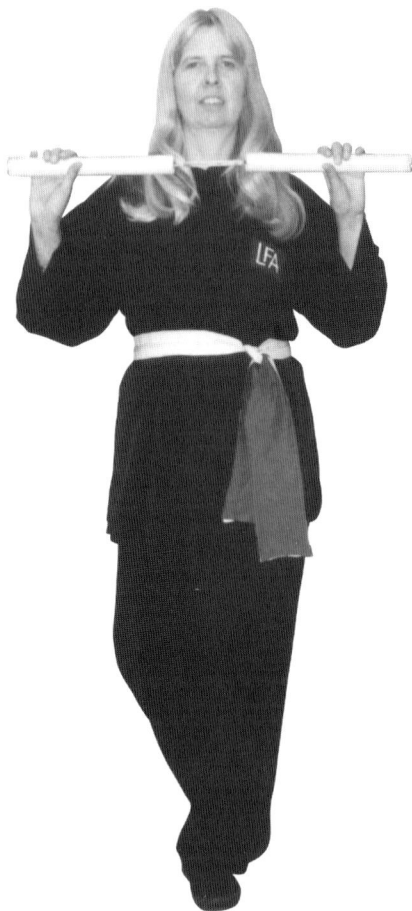

At the same time let go of your nunchaku with your left hand and circle your right hand behind your back transferring your nunchaku from your right hand to your left hand. Now continue the circle with your left hand swinging the free end of your nunchaku round so that you can catch it with your right hand. Your nunchaku finish horizontal at shoulder height.

Note: the photograph shows the front view, but the actual stance is with the back facing the camera.

Number 60

From Right Scissors stance place your right heel down and step sideways (to your left) into Bear stance. This movement is the same as movement number fiftyeight.

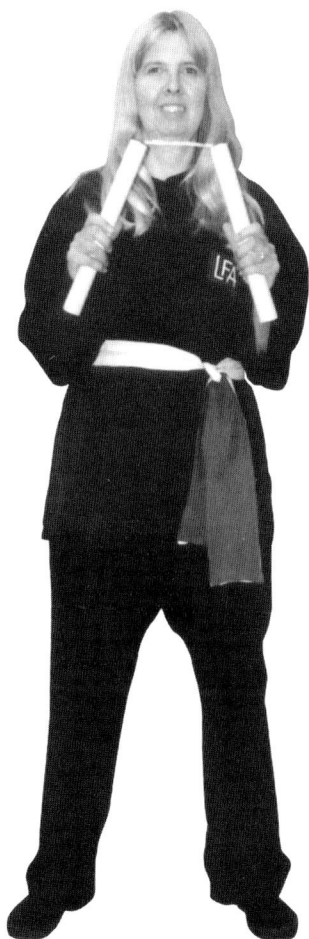

At the same time let go of your nunchaku with your left hand, circle your right hand behind your back, transferring your nunchaku from your right hand to your left hand. Now complete the circle with your left hand swinging the free end round, to be caught by your right hand. The cord is pulled tight, both ends are pointing downwards and slightly inwards towards the body. Note: the photograph shows the front view, but the actual stance is with the back facing the camera.

Number 61

From Bear stance turn ninety degrees to your left into Right Dog stance (bend your left knee to aid your balance).

At the same time move your right hand to your right shoulder (still holding your nunchaku). Your left hand holds the other end which is extended forward at shoulder height (your nunchaku form a straight line).

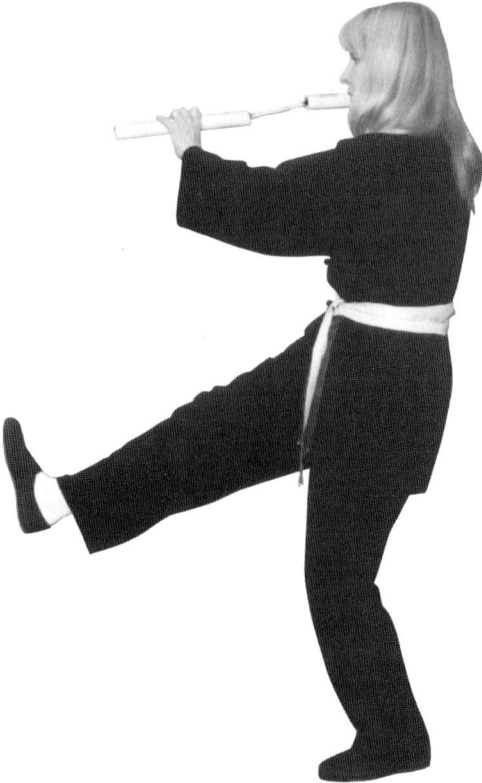

Number 62

From Right Dog bend your right knee into Right Crane stance (your right thigh is parallel to the floor).

At the same time let go of your nunchaku with your left hand. Swing the free end underneath your right leg, catching it with your left hand (cord pulled tight).

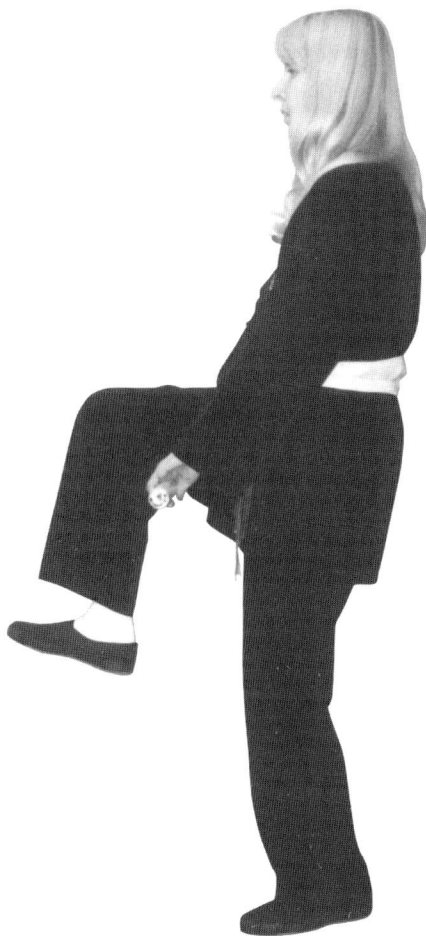

Number 63

From Right Crane stance place your right foot flat on to the floor and raise your left leg into Left Dog stance (bend your right knee to aid your balance).

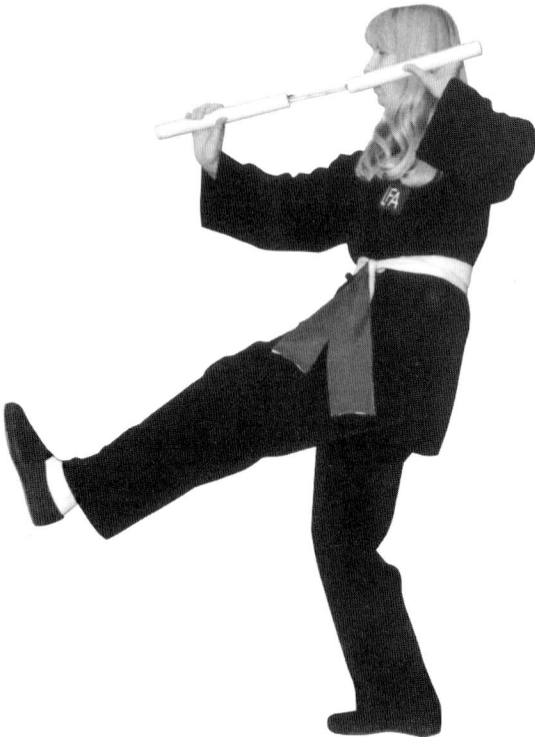

At the same time let go of your nunchaku with your right hand. Pull your nunchaku from underneath your right leg, now move your left hand to your left shoulder. Take hold of the free end of your nunchaku with your right hand, extending it forward at shoulder height (your nunchaku form a straight line).

Number 64

From Left Dog stance bend and raise your left leg into Left Crane stance (left thigh parallel to the floor).

At the same time let go of your nunchaku with your left hand, now swing your nunchaku underneath your left leg catching it with your left hand (cord pulled tight).

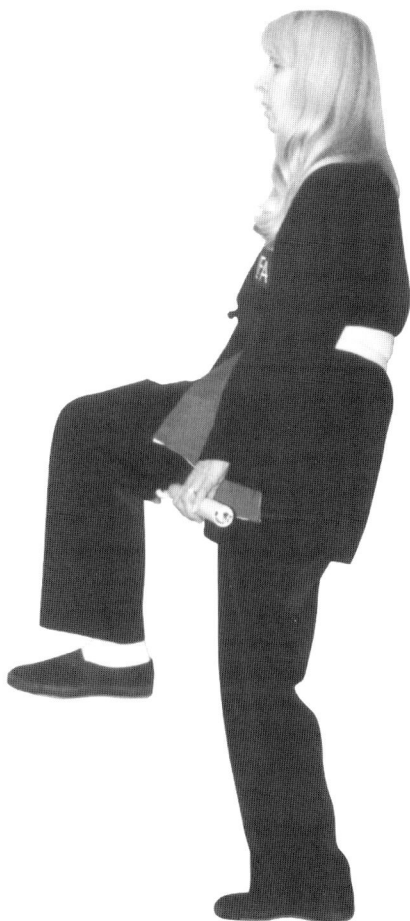

Number 65

From Left Crane stance turn ninety degrees to your left into Right Scissors stance (both knees bent, your right foot is crossed behind your left leg, with the heel raised).

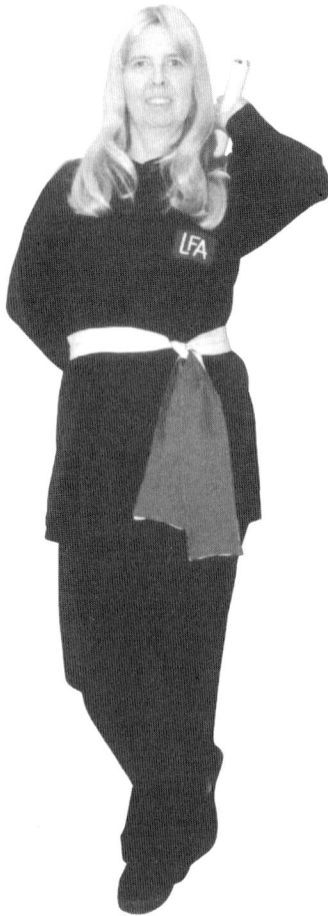

At the same time let go of your nunchaku with your right hand. Swing the free end over your left shoulder, catching it with your right hand behind your back.

Number 66

From Right Scissors stance place your right heel flat on the floor and cross your left foot behind your right leg into Left Scissors stance (both knees are bent, your heel is raised on your left foot.

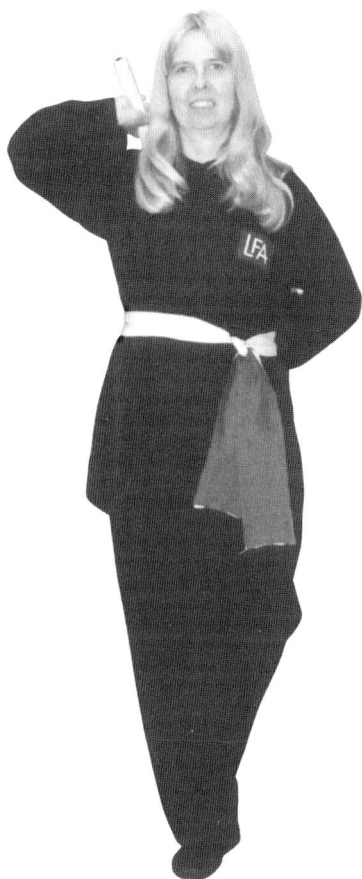

At the same time let go of your nunchaku with your left hand. Swing the free end over your right shoulder, catching it with your left hand behind your back.

Number 67

From Left Scissors stance, step sideways with your left foot into Left Leopard stance (left knee bent, right leg straight).

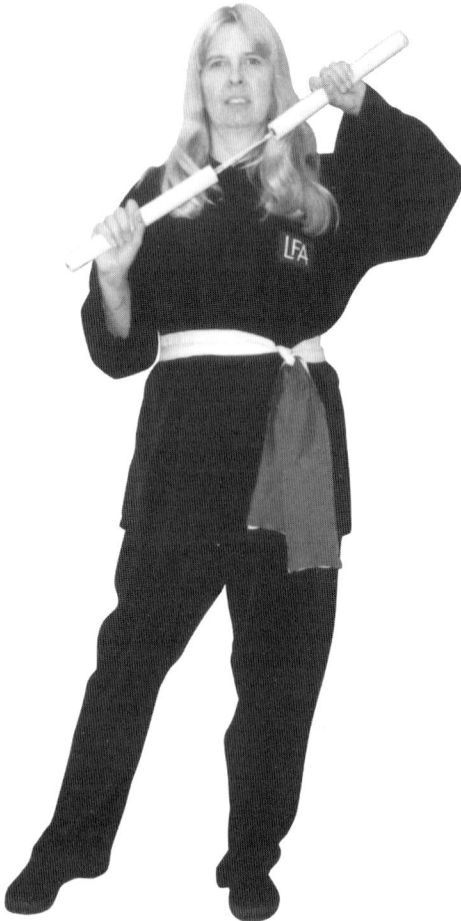

At the same time let go of your nunchaku with your left hand. Swing the free end, downwards then upwards, catching it with your left hand. Your nunchaku are angled downwards from your left shoulder.

Number 68

From Left Leopard stance turn ninety degrees to your left into Right Crane stance (raise and bend your right knee, thigh parallel to the floor).

Your nunchaku finish in the vertical position (left hand high – right hand low.

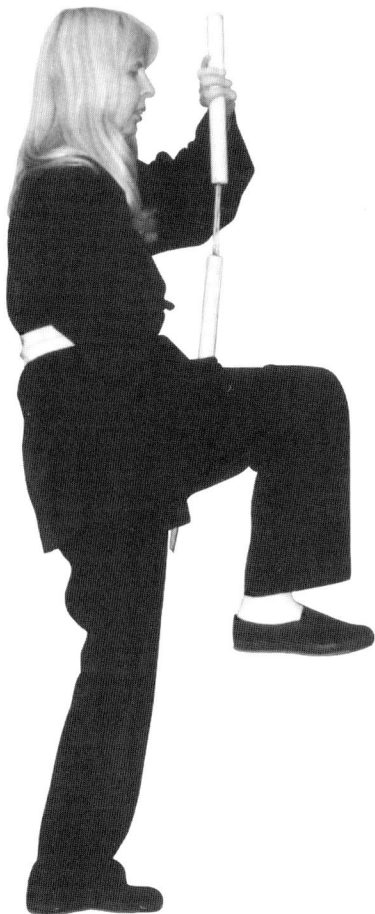

Number 69

From Right Crane stance step behind with your right foot into Left Duck stance (remember to place your right heel down first).

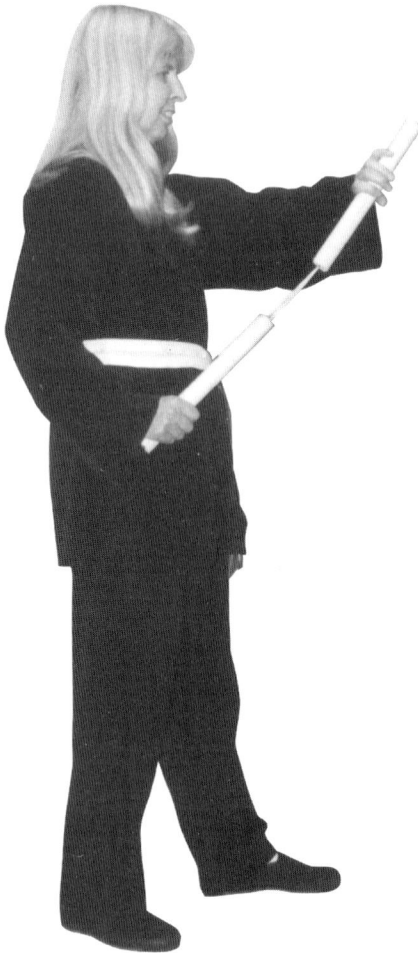

At the same time let go of your nunchaku with your left hand. Circle your right arm up and over (at your right side) so that the free end of your nunchaku is caught with your left hand. Your nunchaku finish angled upwards from your right hip.

Number 70

From Left Duck stance step behind with your left foot into Right Duck stance (remember to place your left heel down first).

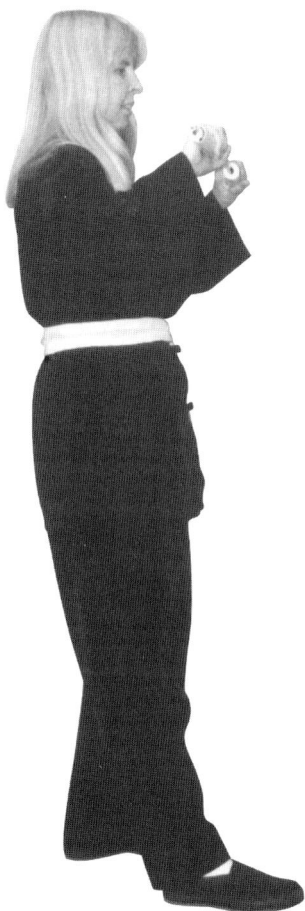

At the same time let go of your nunchaku with your left hand. Circle your right hand behind your back, transferring your nunchaku from right hand to your left hand. Continue the circle, catching the free end with your right hand (finishing with your nunchaku horizontal, at shoulder height).

Number 71

From Right Duck stance turn one hundred and eighty degrees to your right into Right Dragon stance. Remember to apply the principles of the Taoist Walk.

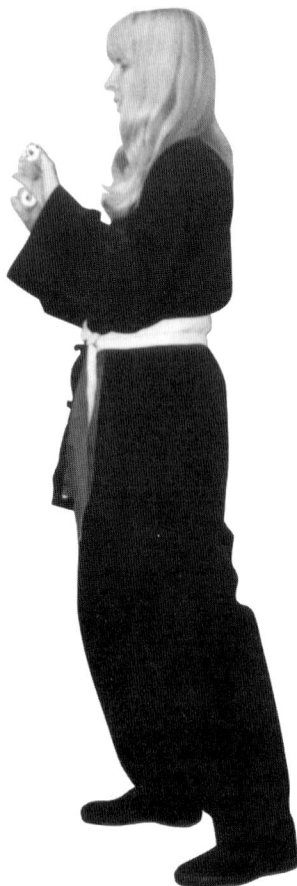

At the same time let go of your nunchaku with your left hand. As you make your turn, circle your nunchaku behind your back, transferring them from your right hand to your left hand. Continue the circle catching the free end with your right hand (finishing with your nunchaku horizontal, at shoulder height).

Number 72

From Right Dragon stance step through into Left Dragon stance. Remember to apply the principles of the Taoist Walk.

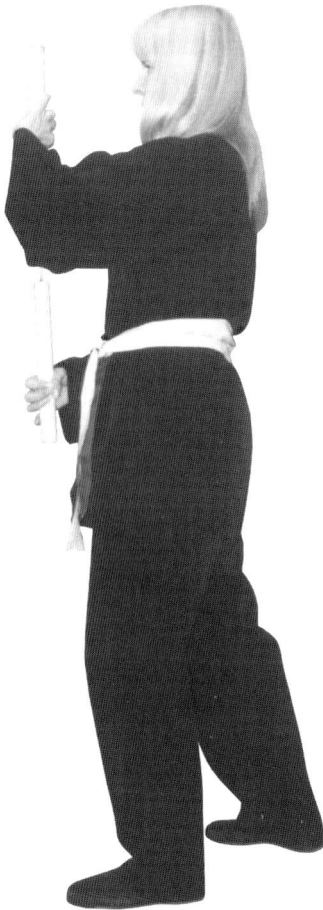

At the same time let go of your nunchaku with your left hand. Circle your right hand behind your back, transferring your nunchaku from your right hand to your left hand. Now pull your n u n c h a k u through, taking hold of the free end with your right hand, so that they finish vertical (left hand high - right hand low).

Number 73

From Left Dragon stance extend your right leg out behind you into Right Hawk stance.
Your nunchaku remain in the same position.

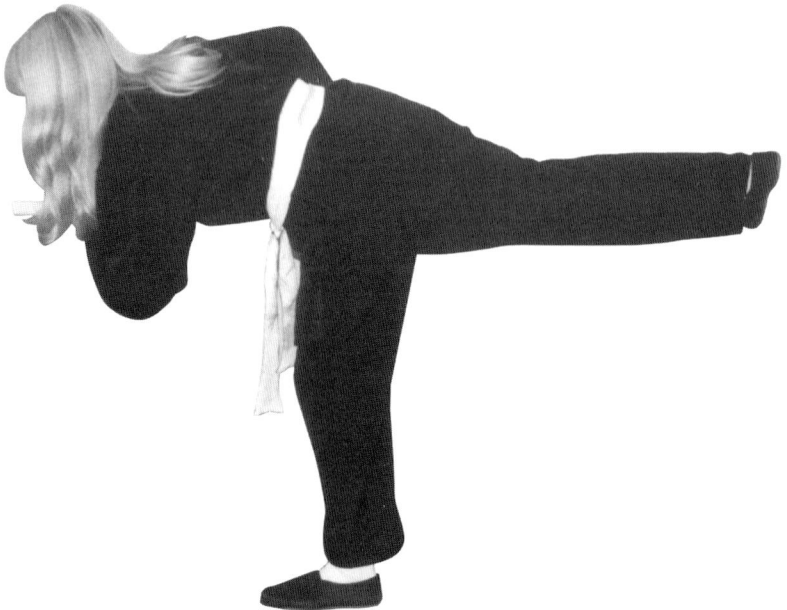

Number 74

From Right Hawk stance step behind with your right foot into Left Duck stance (right knee bent, left leg straight).

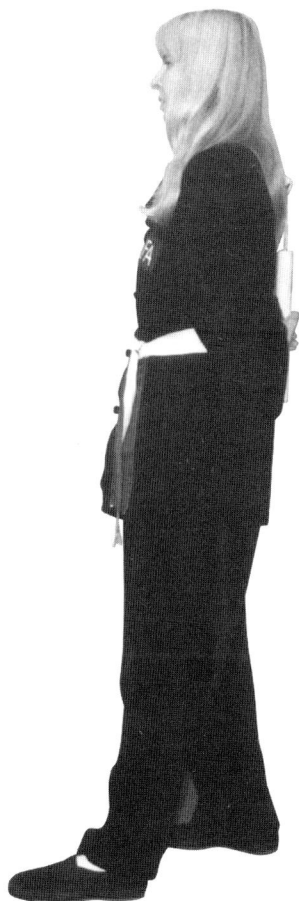

At the same time let go of your nunchaku with your left hand and swing the free end over your right shoulder, catching it behind your back with your left hand.

Number 75

From Left Duck stance step behind with your left foot into Right Duck stance (left knee bent, right leg straight).

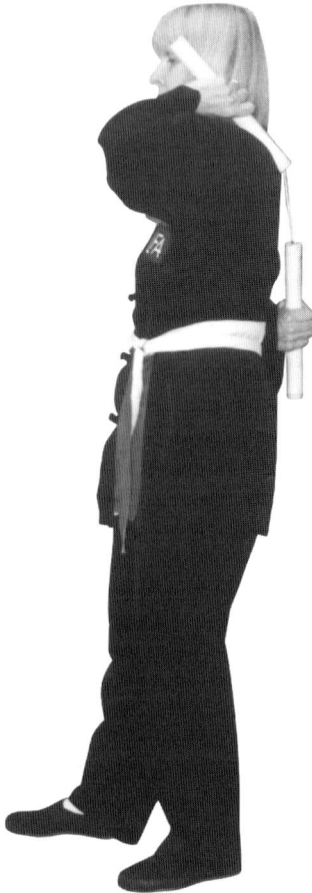

At the same time let go of your nunchaku with your right hand and swing the free end over your left shoulder, catching it behind your back with your right hand.

Number 76

From Right Duck stance turn ninety degrees to your right into Right Leopard stance (right leg bent, left leg straight).

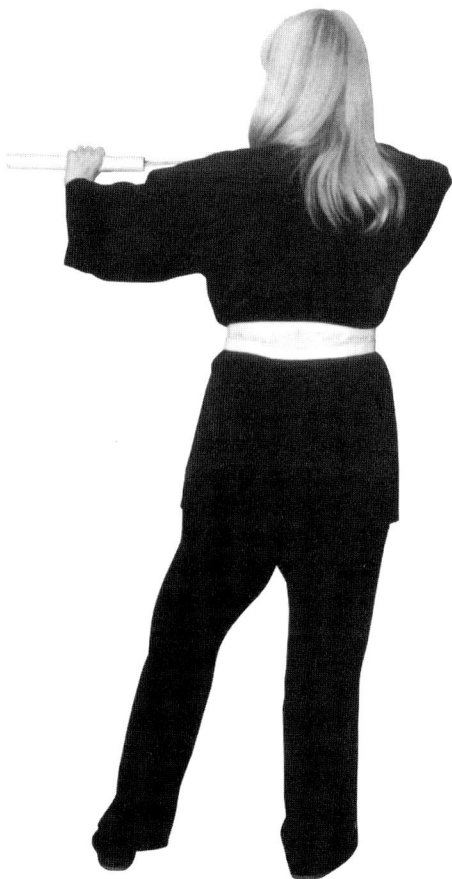

At the same time let go of your nunchaku with your left hand. Circle the free end forwards, then upwards and over to the rear, until you have completed one full circle. Now catch the free end with your left hand so that your nunchaku finish horizontal at shoulder height (extended out to the left hand side of your body, see photograph).

Number 77

From Right Leopard stance cross your right foot behind your left leg into Right Scissors stance (both knees bent, the heel is raised on your right foot).

At the same time centre your nunchaku (see photograph).

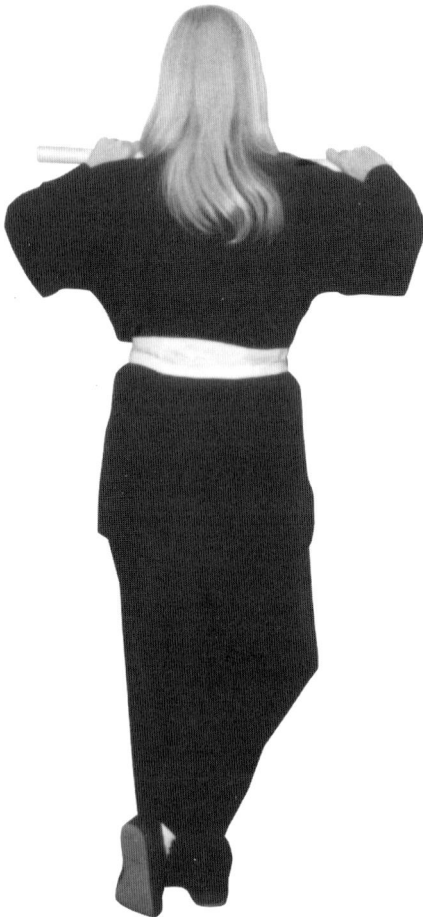

Number 78

From Right Scissors stance turn ninety degrees to your right into Right Dragon stance. Remember to apply the principles of the Taoist Walk.

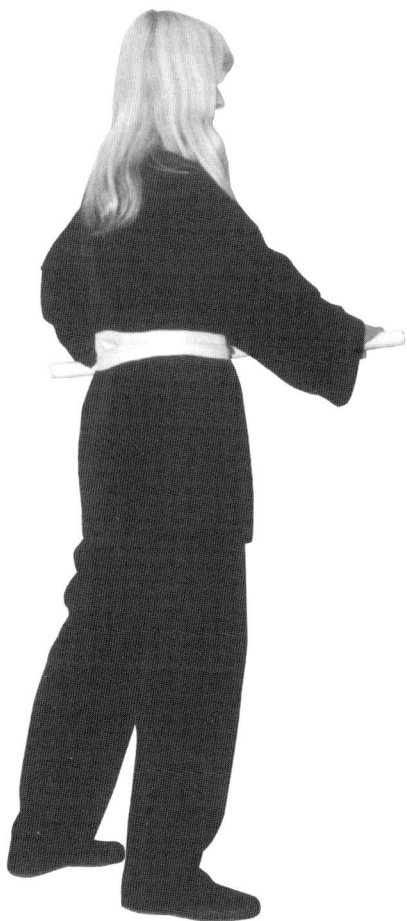

At the same let go of your nunchaku with your left hand and flip the free end over as you make your turn. Catch the free end with your left hand (your n u n c h a k u finish by your left hip, see photograph).

123

Number 79

From Right Dragon stance step through into Left Dragon stance. Remember to apply the principles of the Taoist Walk.

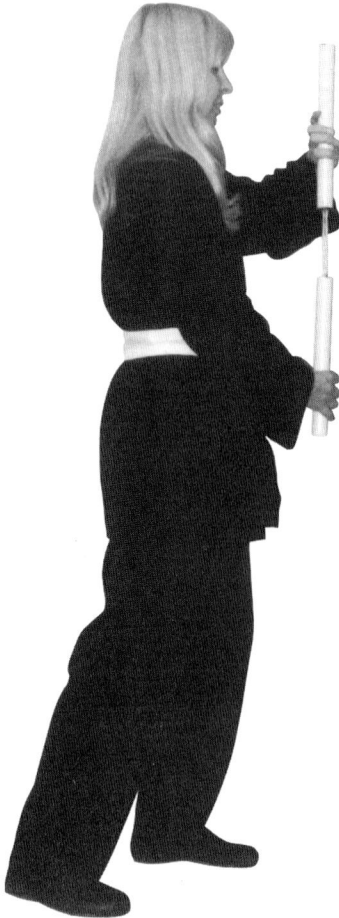

At the same time let go of your nunchaku with your left hand and circle them around your body, transferring your nunchaku from your right hand to your left hand behind your back. Now pull your left hand through so that your nunchaku are now vertical. Take hold of the free end with your right hand (left hand high - right hand low).

Number 80

From Left Dragon stance turn ninety degrees to the right into Right Leopard stance (right knee bent, left leg straight)

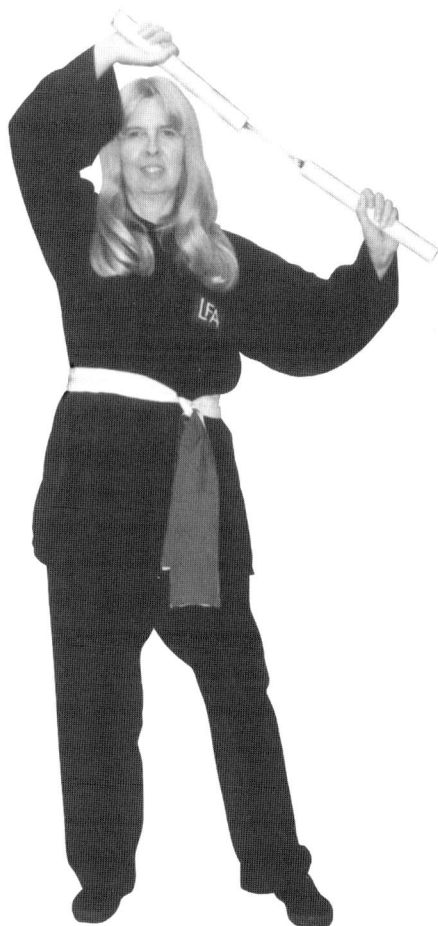

At the same time let go of your nunchaku with your left hand and complete one full circle (circling to the right), then transfer your nunchaku from your right hand to your left hand. Now circle your left hand over to your right, transfer your nunchaku from your left hand to your right hand. Now catch the free end of your nunchaku with your left hand, finishing with your nunchaku angled downwards from right to left.

Number 81

From Right Leopard stance cross your right foot behind your left leg into Right Scissors stance (both knees bent, your heel is raised on your right foot).

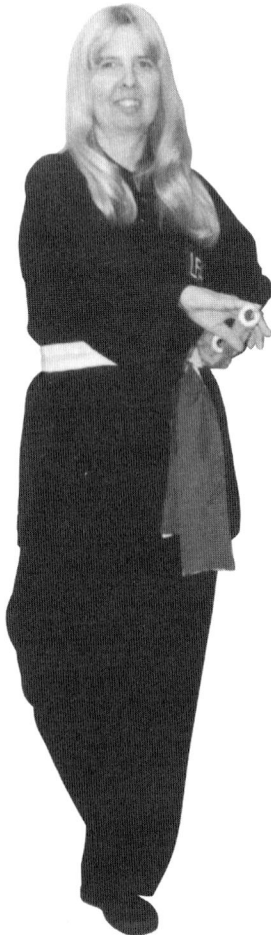

At the same time let go of your nunchaku with your left hand. Now flip the free end of your nunchaku over, catching it with your left hand near to your left hip (see photograph).

Number 82

From Right Scissors stance raise your right leg into Right Stork stance (bend your left knee to aid your balance).

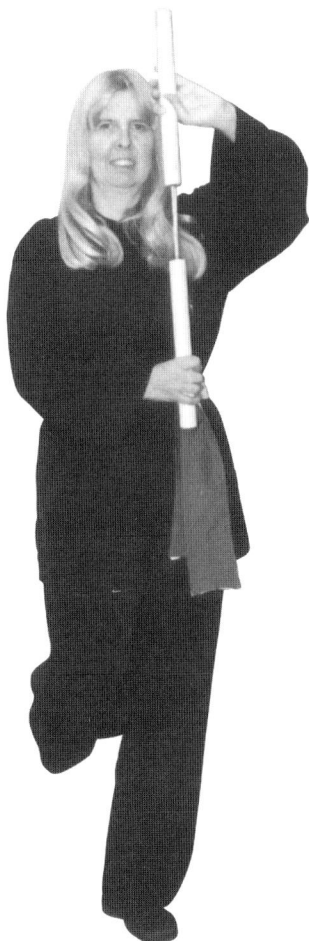

At the same time let go of your nunchaku with your left hand. Circle them round your body, transferring them from your right hand to your left hand behind your back. Circle your left hand round to the front of your body, taking hold of the free end with your right hand. Your nunchaku finish vertical, left hand high - right hand low).

Number 83

From Right Stork stance turn ninety degrees to your right into Right Dragon stance. Remember to apply the principles of the Taoist Walk.

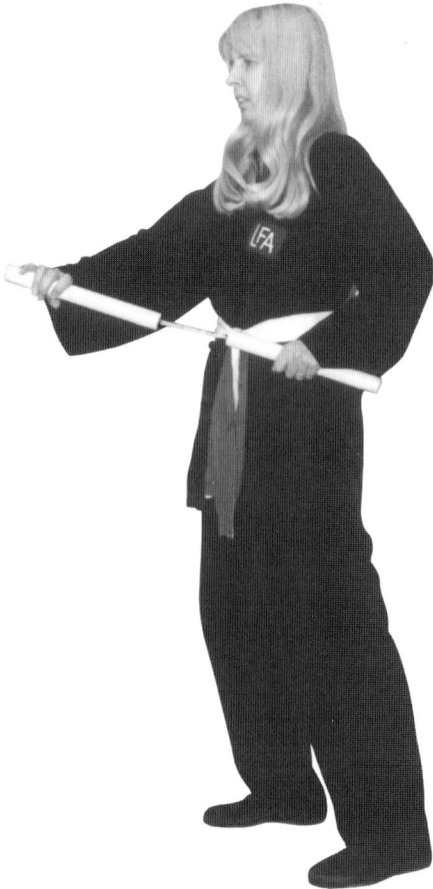

At the same time let go of your nunchaku with your left hand. Now flip the free end over catching it with your left hand by your left hip, (the nunchaku are angled upwards from your left hip).

Number 84

From Right Dragon stance step through into Left Dragon stance. Remember to apply the principles of the Taoist Walk.

At the same time let go of your nunchaku with your right hand. Now flip the free end over, catching it with your right hand by your right hip, (your nunchaku finish angled upwards from your right hip).

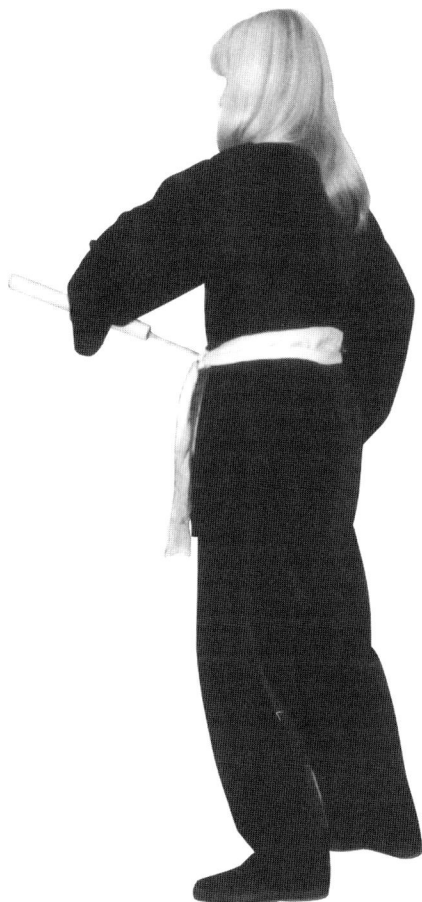

Number 85

From Left Dragon stance step behind with your left foot into Right Duck stance (left knee bent, right leg straight).

At the same time let go of your nunchaku with your left hand. Swing the free end over your right shoulder, catching it behind your back with your left hand.

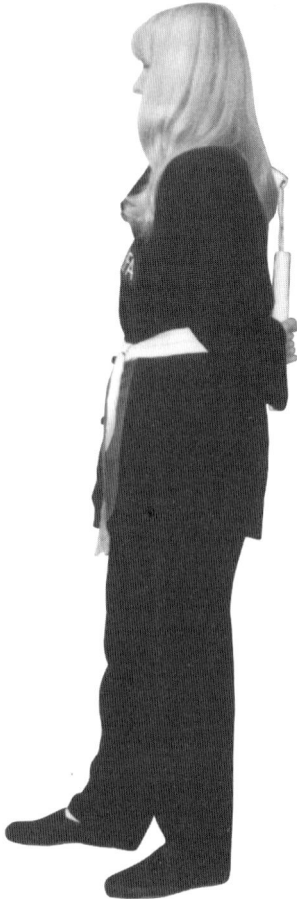

Number 86

From Right Duck stance turn one hundred and eighty degrees to your left into Left Dragon stance.

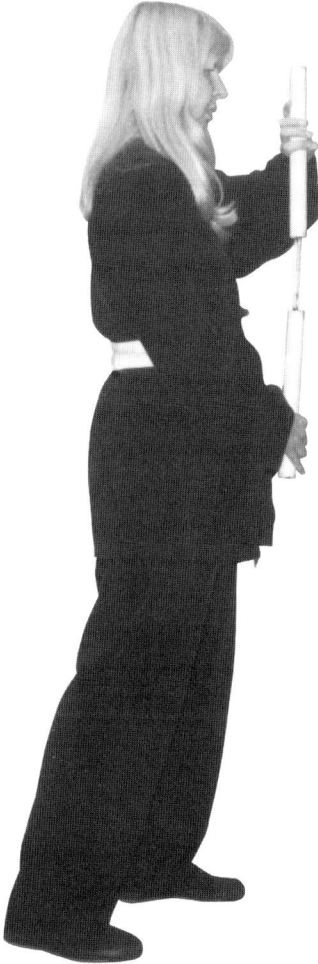

At the same time let go of your nunchaku with your right hand. Move your left hand round to the front of your body. Your nunchaku finish vertical (left hand high - right hand low.

Number 87

From Left Dragon stance turn ninety degrees to your left into Right Stork stance (bend your left knee to aid your balance).

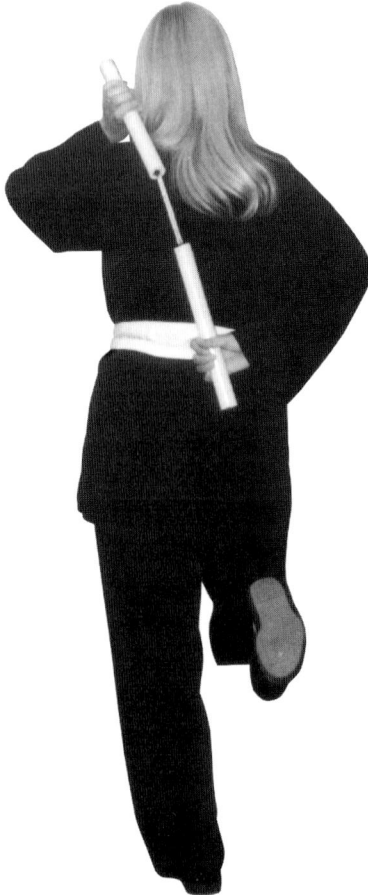

At the same time let go of your nunchaku with your right hand. Swing the free end over your left shoulder, catching it with your right hand behind your back.

Number 88

From Right Stork stance turn one hundred and eighty degrees to your right into Riding Horse stance.

At the same time let go of your nunchaku with your right hand. Circle your nunchaku around the front of your body, then transfer them from your left hand to your right hand. Continue circling your nunchaku round transferring them from your right hand to your left hand behind your back, finally catching the free end with your right hand in front of your body (at shoulder height).

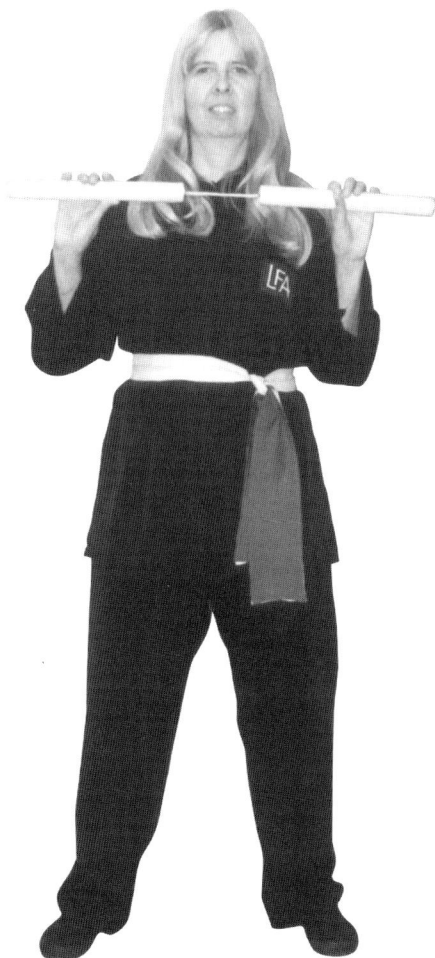

Number 89

From Riding Horse stance turn fortyfive degrees to your right into Right Crane stance (raise and bend your right knee, your right thigh is parallel to the floor).

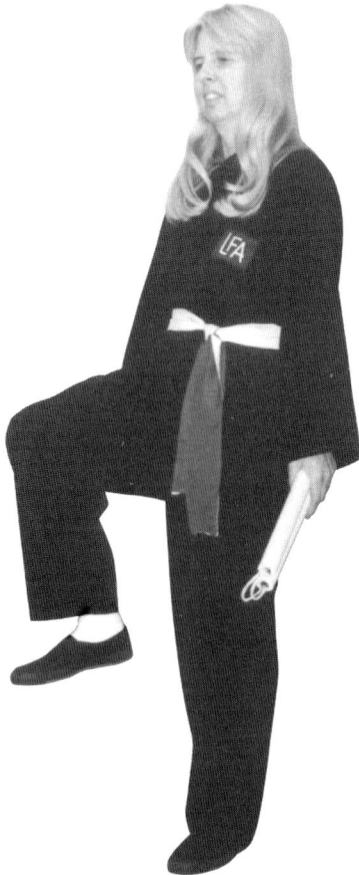

At the same time let go of your nunchaku with your right hand, flip the free end forwards and over and back towards you, catching it with your left hand (both ends of your nunchaku are now in your left hand).

Number 90

From Right Crane stance place your right foot flat on the floor and raise your left leg into Left Crane stance. At the same time flip one end of your nunchaku forwards, over and back towards you, simultaneously exchange the end of your nunchaku in your left hand to your right hand and catch the free end of your nunchaku also in your right hand. Both ends of your nunchaku should now be in your right hand.

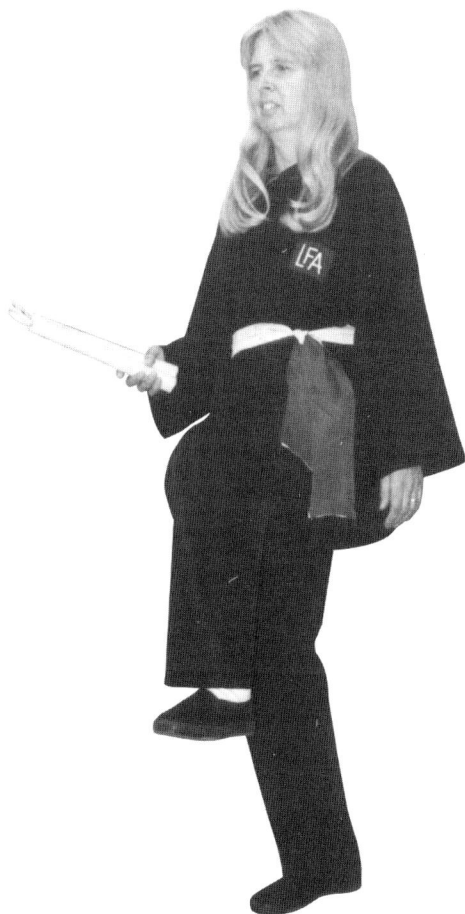

Number 91

From Left Crane stance turn one hundred and thirty five degrees to your left into Left Dragon stance. Remember to apply the principles of the Taoist Walk.

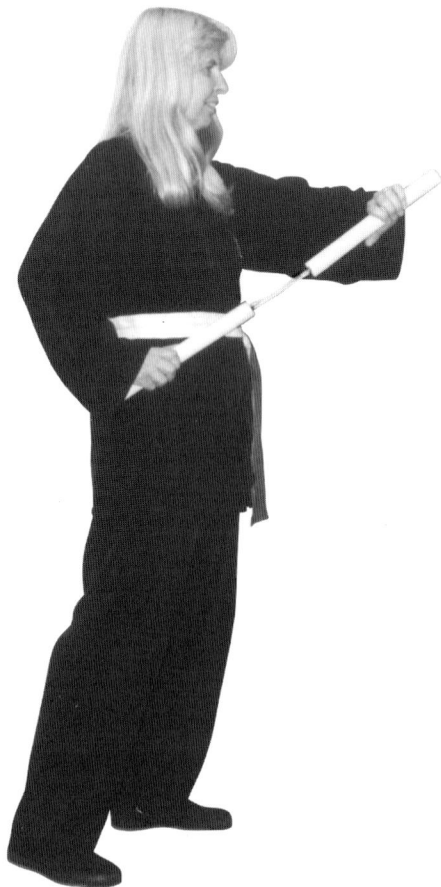

At the same time as you make your turn let go of one end of your nunchaku and circle your right hand, behind your back, exchange your nunchaku from your right hand to your left hand. Now catch the free end with your right hand by your right hip (your nunchaku finish angled upwards from your right hip.

Number 92

From Left Dragon stance raise your right leg out behind you into Right Hawk stance.

At the same time keep hold of your nunchaku with both hands and simply bring your left hand into alignment with your right hand.

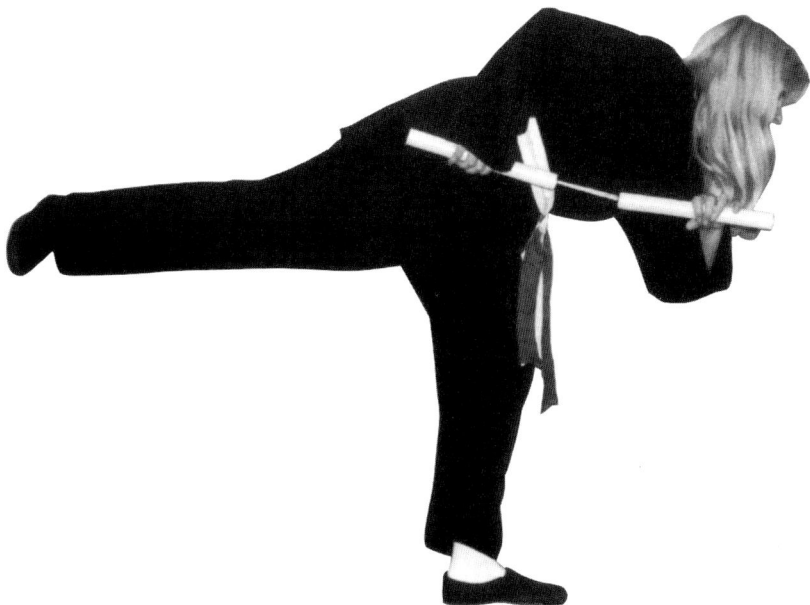

Number 93

From Right Hawk stance swing your right leg forwards into Right Dog stance.

At the same time swing your left hand onto your left shoulder, your right hand follows the movement of the left (see photograph).

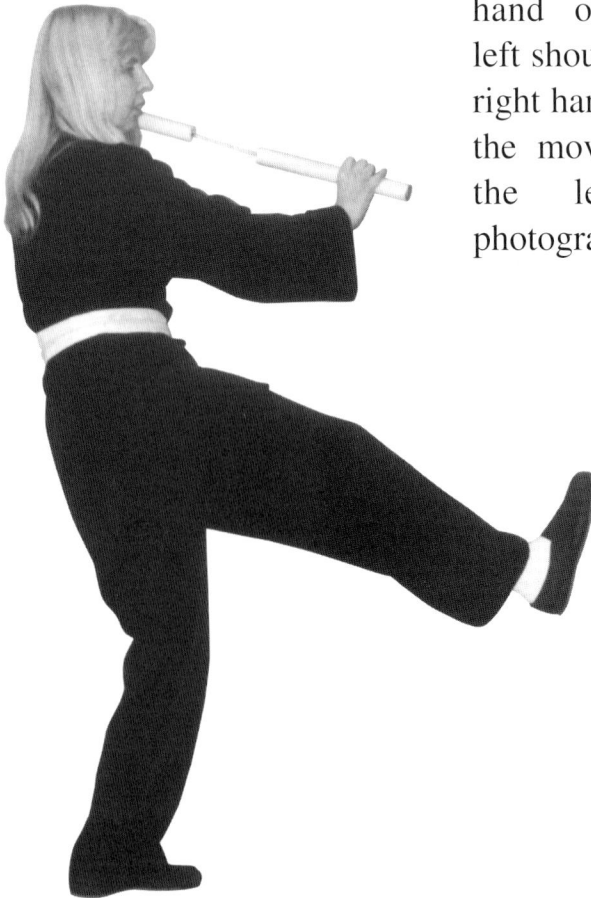

Number 94

From Right Dog stance step through into Right Dragon stance. Remember to apply the principles of the Taoist Walk.

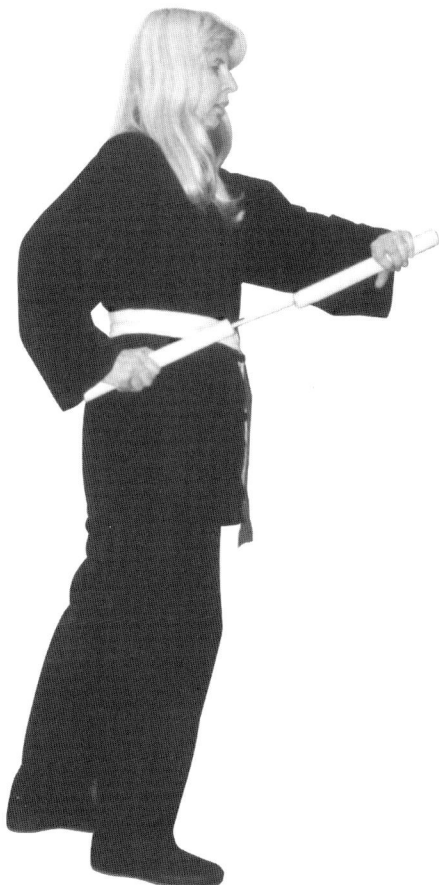

At the same time (still holding onto your nunchaku with both hands), circle your left hand over the top until your right hand is by your right hip (your nunchaku finish angled upwards from your right hip).

Number 95

From Right Dragon stance draw your right foot into Right Snake stance.

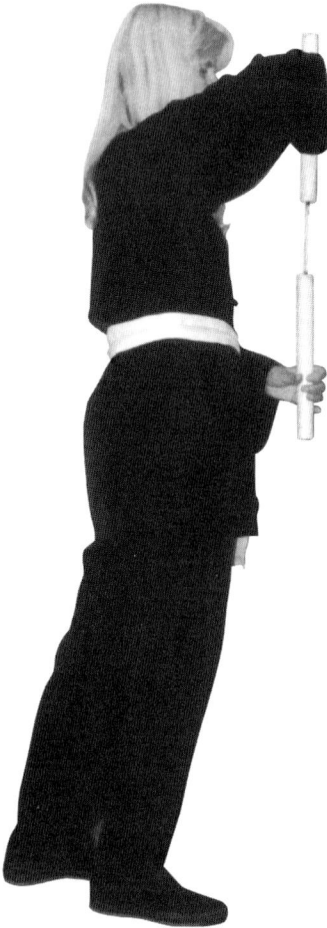

At the same time (still holding your nunchaku with both hands), turn your left hand downwards and your right hand upwards so that your nunchaku are vertical.

Number 96

From Right Snake stance turn ninety degrees to your left into Left Leopard stance (left knee bent, right leg straight).

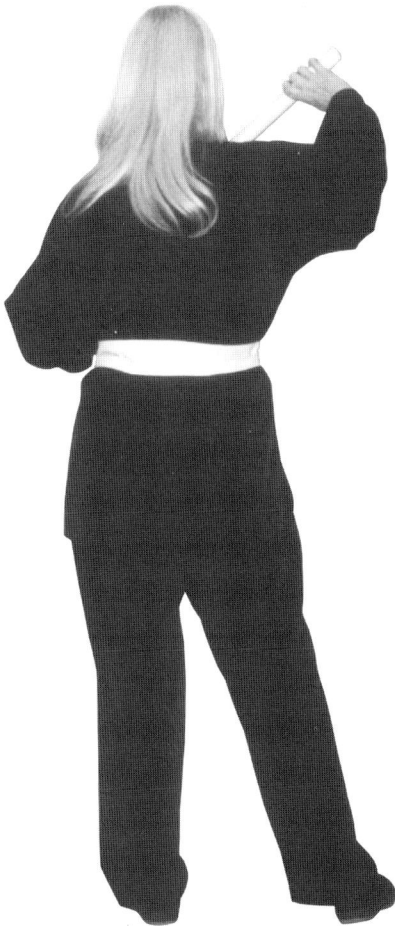

At the same time let go of your nunchaku with your right hand and circle your left hand to the left, swinging the free end of your nunchaku across to your right. Catch the free end with your right hand, your nunchaku finish angled downwards from right to left.

Number 97

From Left Leopard stance raise your right leg into Right Crane stance (right knee bent, your right thigh is parallel to the floor).

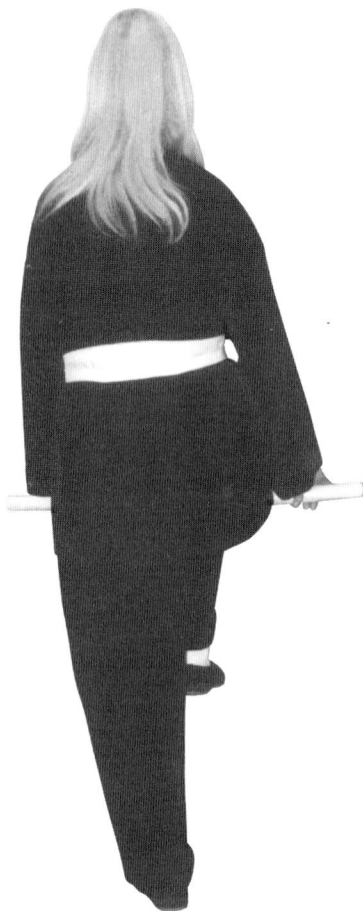

At the same time let go of your nunchaku with your left hand. Swing the free end of your nunchaku underneath your right leg, catching it with your left hand (cord pulled tight).

Number 98

From Right Crane stance cross your right foot behind your left leg into Right Scissors stance (both knees are bent, the heel is raised on your right foot).

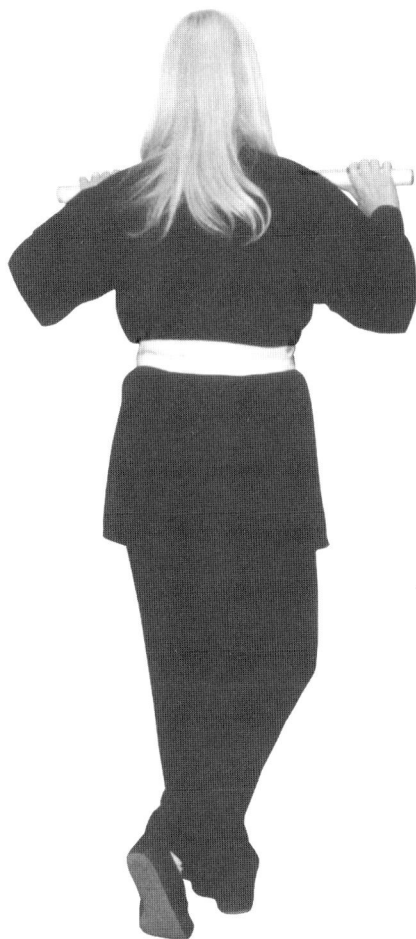

At the same time let go of your nunchaku with your right hand. Circle your nunchaku around in front of your body, transferring them from your left hand to your right hand, then from your right hand to your left hand (behind your back), finally catching the free end in front of your body with your right hand (at shoulder height).

Number 99

From Right Scissors stance turn ninety degrees to your left into Left Dragon stance. Remember to apply the principles of the Taoist Walk.

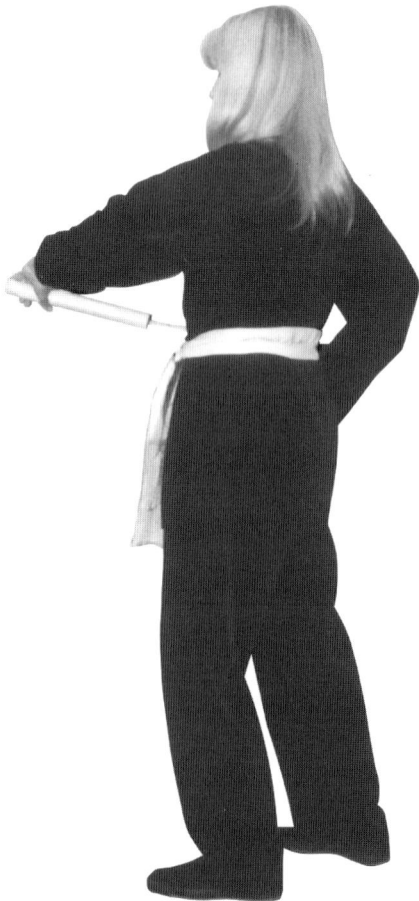

At the same time let go of your nunchaku with your right hand, flip the free end over catching it with your right hand by your right hip.

Number 100

From Left Dragon stance raise your left leg into Left Crane stance (left knee bent, thigh parallel to the floor).

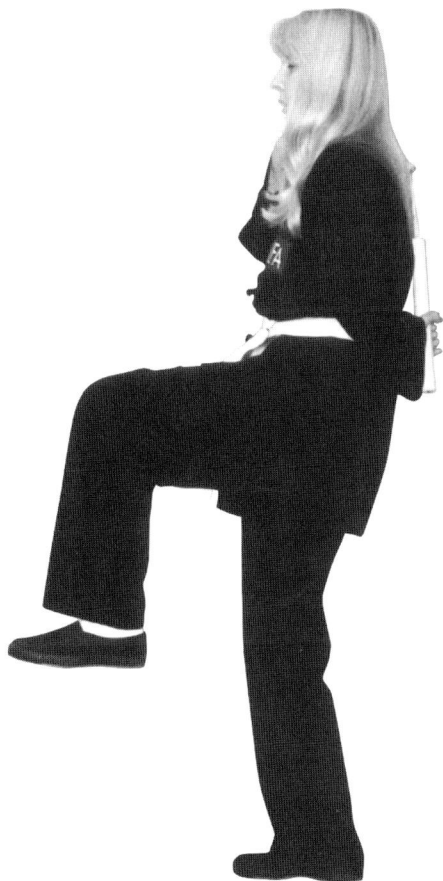

At the same time let go of your nunchaku with your left hand and swing the free end over your right shoulder catching it behind your back with your left hand.

Number 101

From Left Crane stance turn ninety degrees to your left into Right Scissors stance (both knees bent, the heel is raised on your right foot).

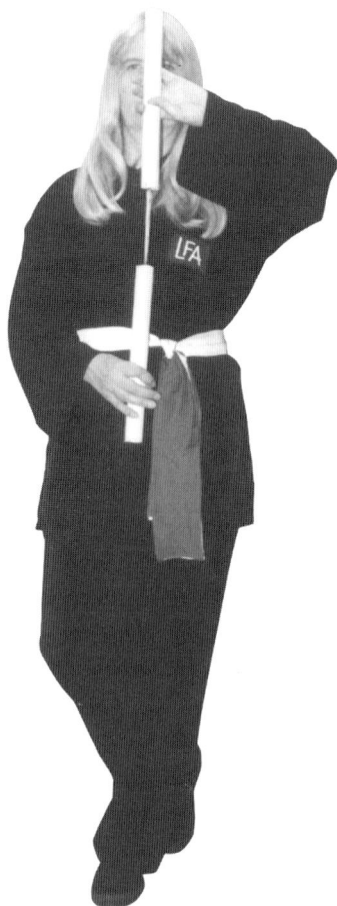

At the same time let go of your nunchaku with your left hand. Move your right hand over the top (forwards), then transfer your nunchaku from your right hand to your left hand. Now take hold of the free end of your nunchaku with your right hand. Your nunchaku finish vertical left hand high – right hand low.

Number 102

From Right Scissors stance step sideways with your left foot into Left Leopard stance (left knee bent, right leg straight).

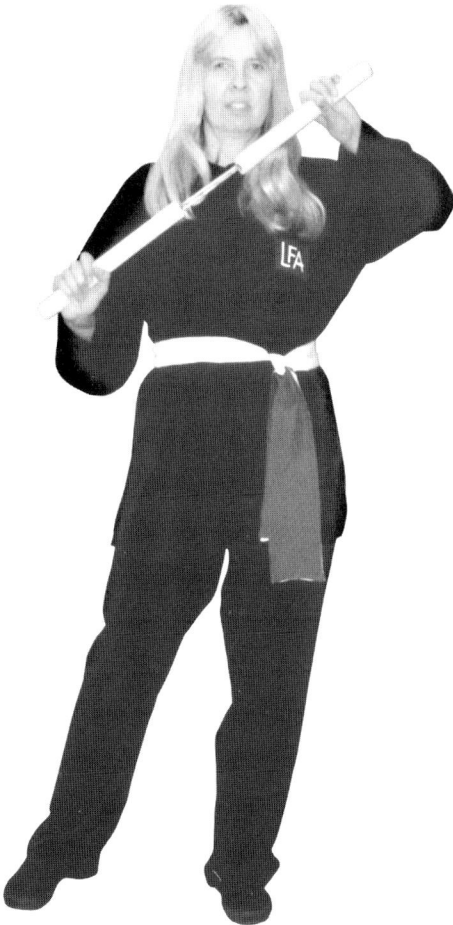

At the same move your left hand to your left shoulder. Your nunchaku finish angled d o w n w a r d from left to right.

Number 103

From Left Leopard stance cross your right foot in front of your left leg into Right Crossed Legs stance (both knees bent, your heel is raised on your right foot).

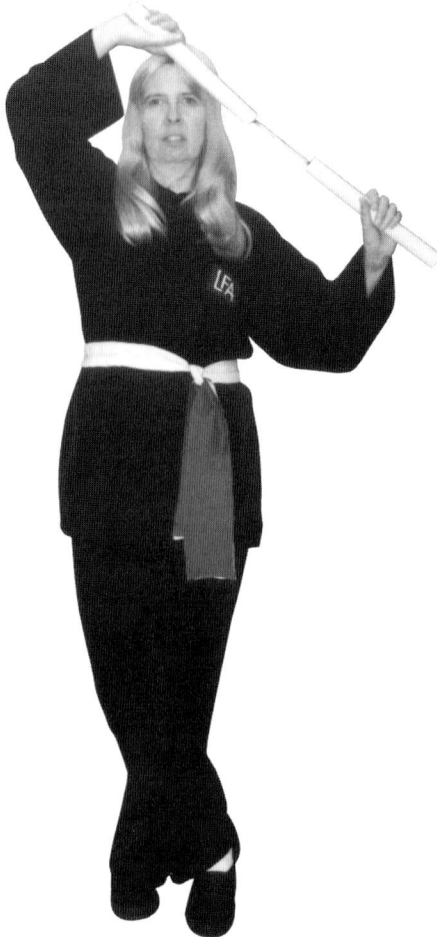

At the same time let go of your nunchaku with your left hand and circle them to your right, catching the free end with your left hand. Your nunchaku finish angled downwards from right to left.

LFA T'AI CHI NUNCHAKU

Number 104

From Right Crossed Legs stance turn ninety degrees to your left into Left Dragon stance. Remember to apply the principles of the Taoist Walk.

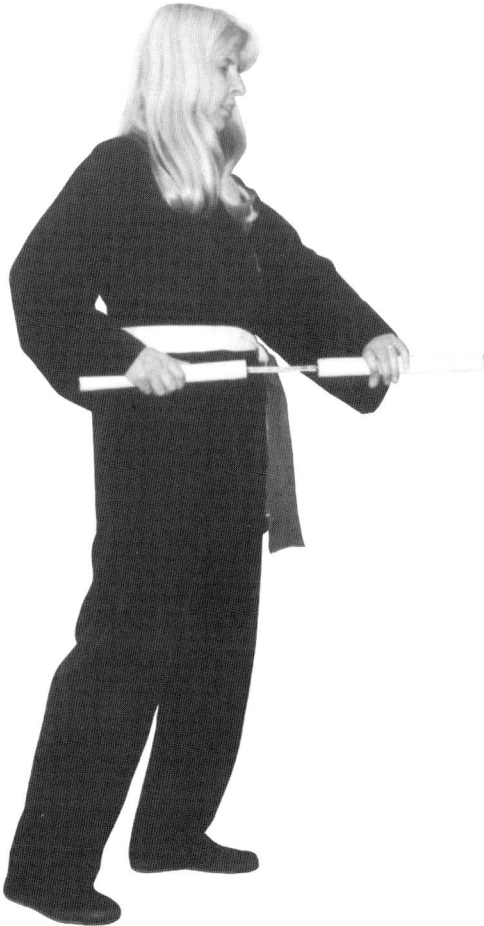

At the same time let go of your nunchaku with your right hand. Flip your nunchaku forwards and catch the free end with your right hand near your right hip.

Number 105

From Left Dragon stance raise your right leg out behind you into Right Hawk stance.

Your nunchaku remain in the same position as they were in for movement number one hundred and four.

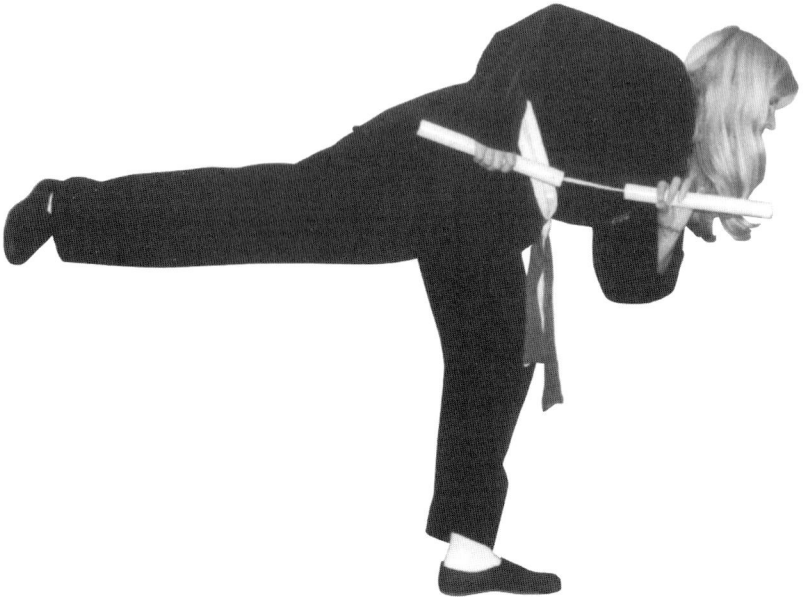

Number 106

From Right Hawk stance swing your right leg through into Right Dog stance.

At the same time move your left hand onto your right shoulder. Your right hand moves forward with the movement of the left.

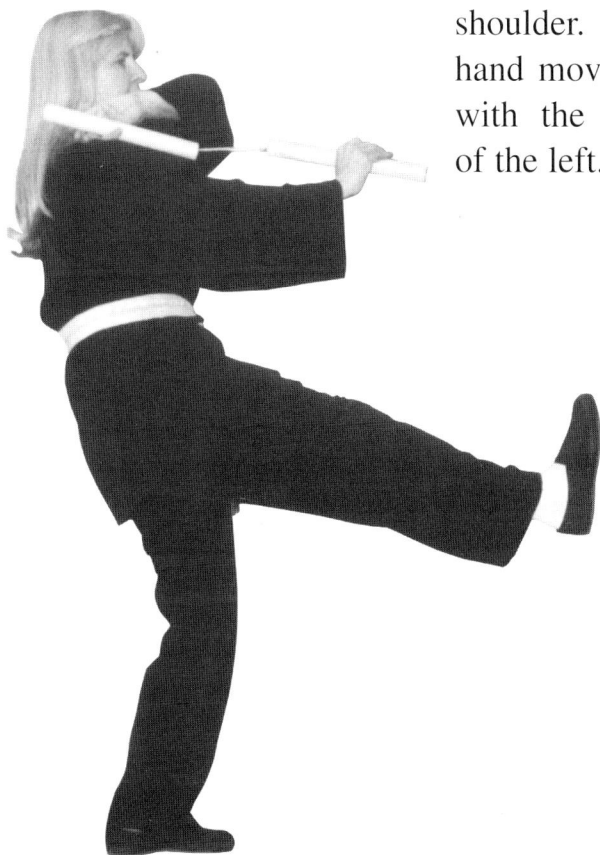

Number 107

From Right Dog stance lower your leg into Right Dragon stance.

At the same time move both hands so that your nunchaku are horizontal at s h o u l d e r height.

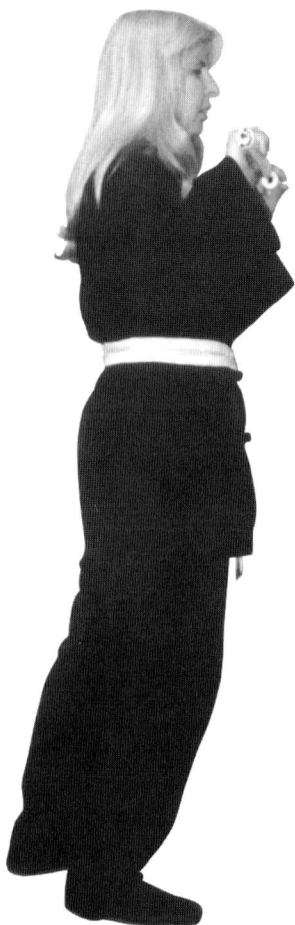

Number 108

From Right Dragon stance turn ninety degrees to your left into Right Scissors stance (both knees bent, the heel is raised on your right foot).

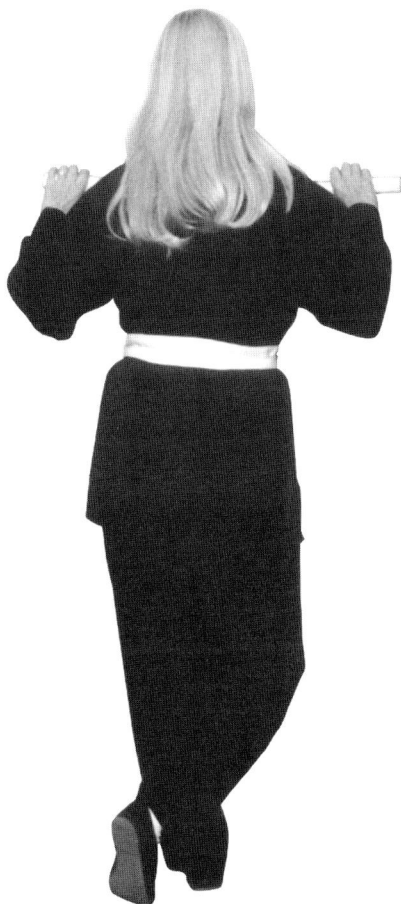

At the same time let go of your nunchaku with your right hand. Now flip the free end to the left and catch it with your right hand. Your nunchaku finish horizontal at shoulder height.

Number 109

From Right Crossed Legs stance turn ninety degrees to your left into Left Dragon stance.

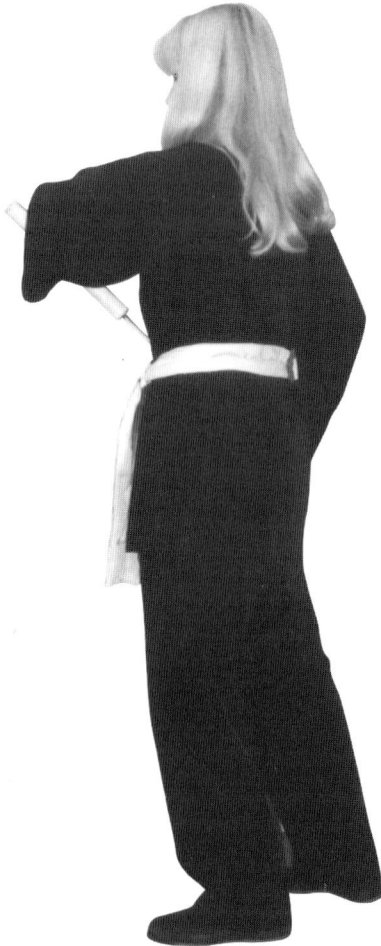

At the same time let go your nunchaku with your right hand. Flip your nunchaku forwards catching the free end with your right hand. Your nunchaku finish angled upwards from your right hip.

Number 110

From Left Dragon stance step behind with your left foot into Right Duck stance (left knee bent, right leg straight).

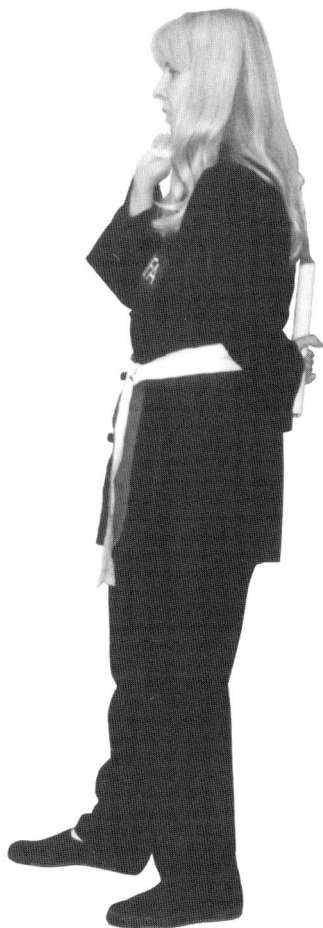

At the same time let go of your nunchaku with your left hand and swing the free end over your right shoulder, catching it behind your back with your left hand.

Number 111

From Right Duck stance step behind with your right foot into Left Duck stance (remember to put your right heel down first).

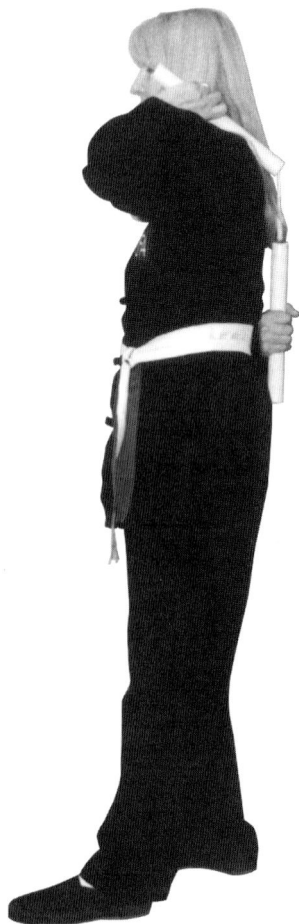

At the same time let go of your nunchaku with your right hand and swing the free end over your left shoulder, catching it behind your back with your right hand.

Number 112

From Left Duck stance turn one hundred and eighty degrees to your right into Right Dragon stance. Remember to apply the principles of the Taoist Walk.

At the same time let go of your nunchaku with your left hand and move the free end round to the front of your body with your right hand. Take hold of the free end with your left hand. Your nunchaku finish vertical, right hand high - left hand low.

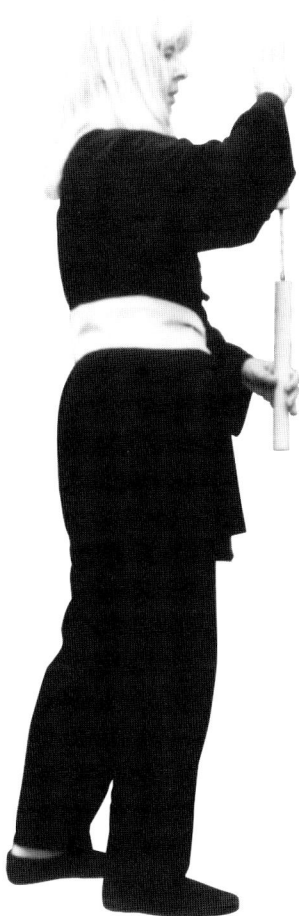

Number 113

From Right Dragon stance turn ninety degrees to your right into Left Scissors stance (both knees bent, the heel is raise on your left foot.)

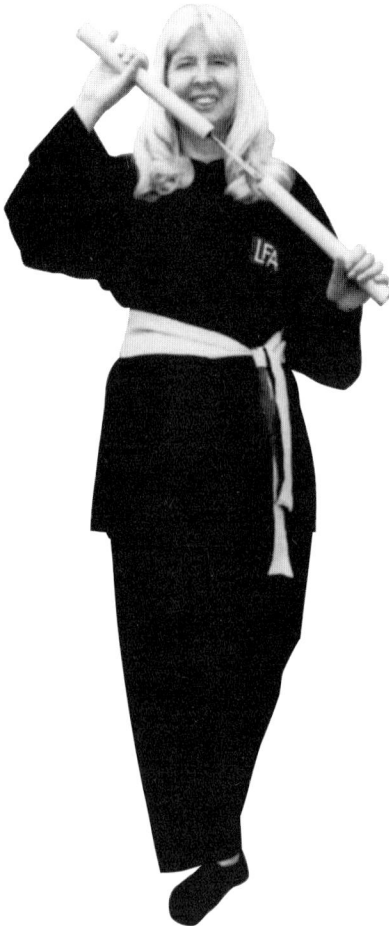

At the same time let go of your nunchaku with your left hand. Flip your nunchaku to the right, swing the free end over and catch it with your left hand. Your nunchaku finish angled down from right to left.

Number 114

From Left Scissors stance step sideways into Right Leopard stance (right leg bent, left leg straight).

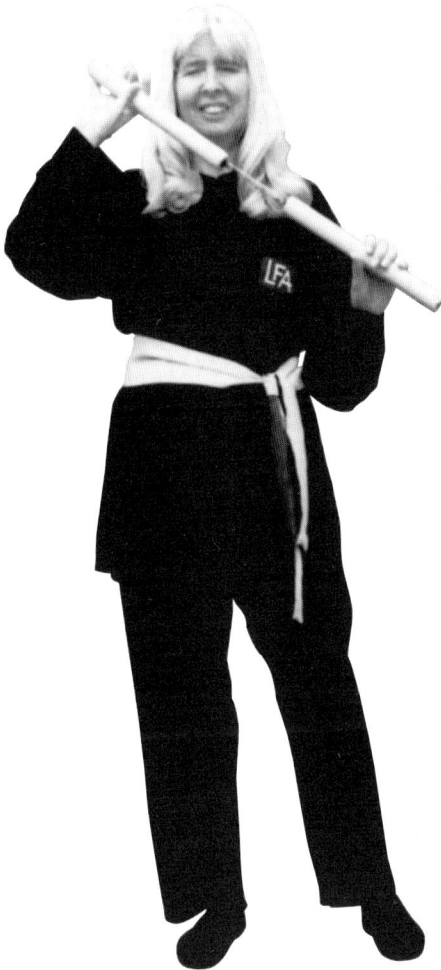

Your nunchaku remain in the same position as they were in for movement one hundred and thirteen.

Number 115

From Right Leopard stance raise your left leg into Left Stork stance.

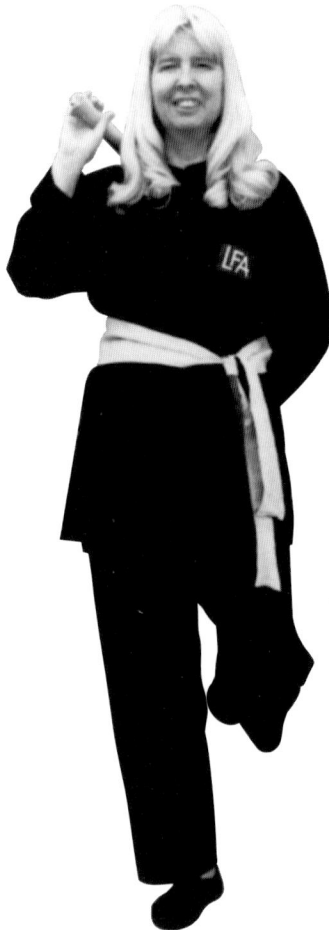

At the same time let go of your nunchaku with your left hand and swing the free end over your right shoulder catching it behind your back with your left hand.

Number 116

From Left Stork stance cross your left foot in front of your right leg into Left Crossed Legs stance (both knees bent, the heel is raised on your left foot).

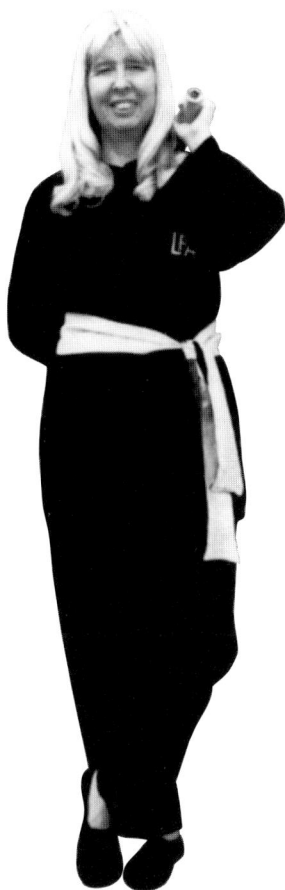

At the same time let go of your nunchaku with your right hand and swing the free end over your left shoulder. Catch the free end behind your back with your right hand.

Number 117

From Left Crossed Legs stance turn ninety degrees to your right into Right Dragon stance.

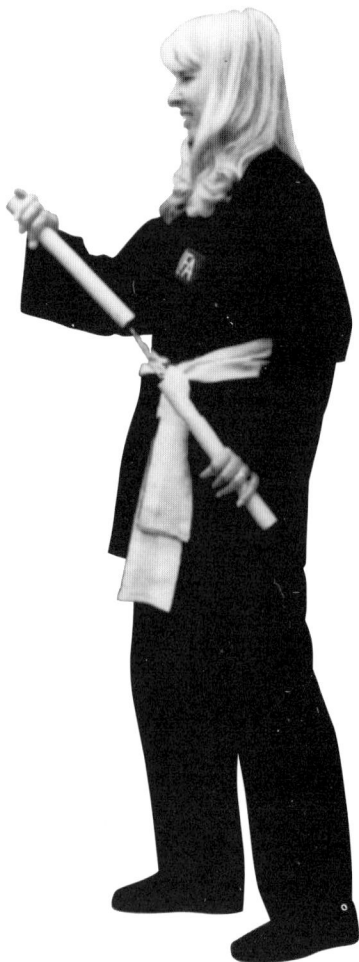

At the same time let go of your nunchaku with your left hand. Pull the free end of your nunchaku through and circle it round to catch it with your left hand by your left hip. Your nunchaku finish angled upwards from your left hip.

Number 118

From Right Dragon stance step through into Left Dragon stance. Remember to apply the principles of the Taoist Walk.

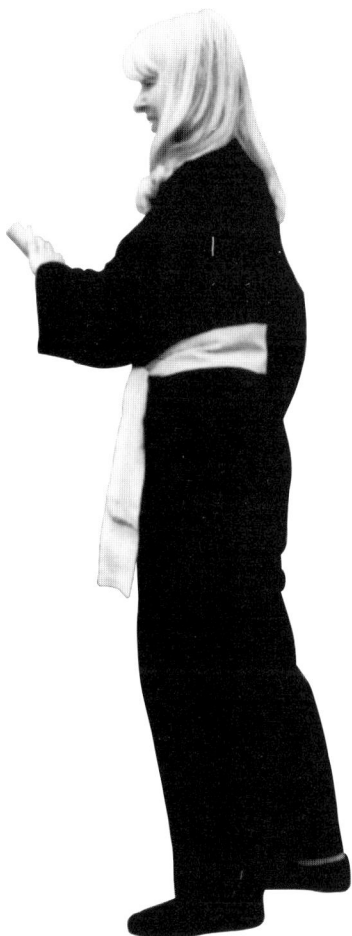

At the same time let go of your nunchaku with your right hand. Swing the free end of your nunchaku over to the right side of your body, catching it with your right hand near to your right hip. Your nunchaku finish angled upwards from your right hip.

Number 119

From Left Dragon stance step through into Right Dragon stance. Remember to apply the principles of the Taoist Walk.

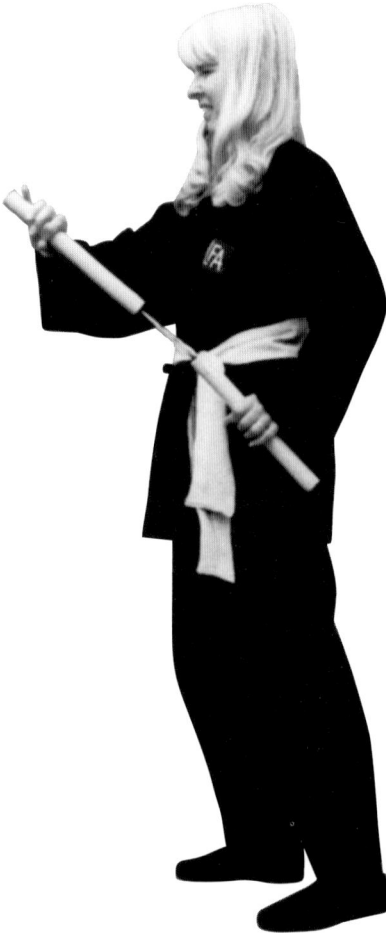

At the same time let go of your nunchaku with your left hand, swing the free end of your nunchaku across to your left side, catching it with your left hand. Your nunchaku finish angled upwards from your left hip.

Number 120

From Right Dragon stance step through into Left Dragon stance. Remember to apply the principles of the Taoist Walk.

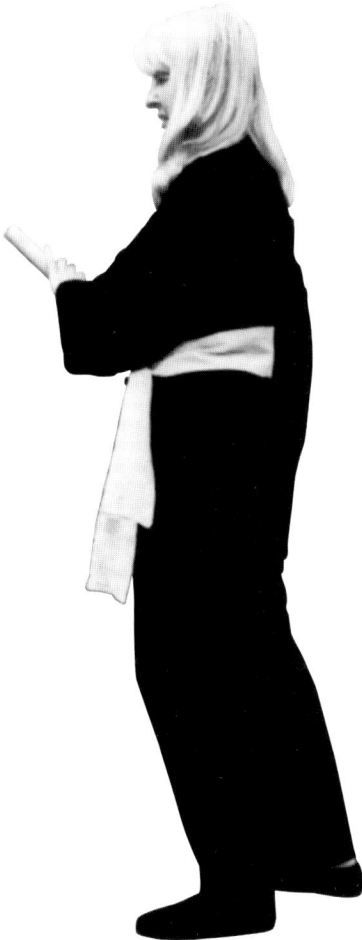

At the same time let go of your nunchaku with your right hand and swing the free end across to the right, catching it with your right hand. Your nunchaku finish angled upwards from your right hip.

Number 121

From Left Dragon stance turn one hundred and eighty degrees to the right into Right Dragon. Remember to apply the principles of the Taoist Walk.

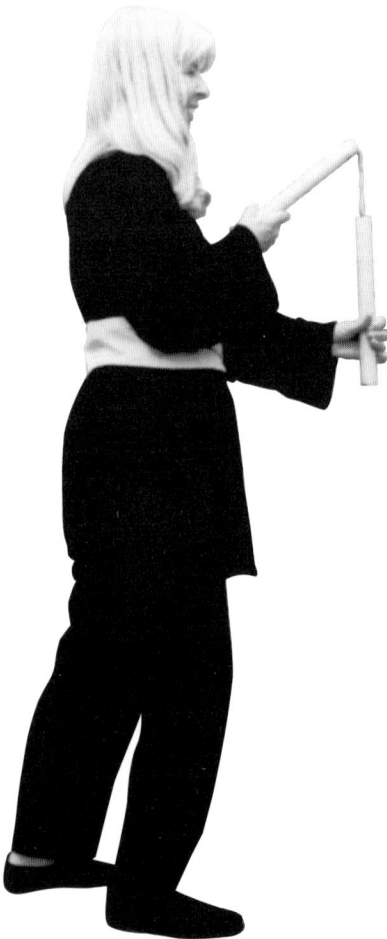

At the same time let go of your nunchaku with your left hand. Your right hand comes over the top as you make your turn, finishing extended forwards at shoulder height. Take hold of the free end of your nunchaku with your left hand; to finish like movement number twenty.

Number 122

From Right Dragon stance step behind with your right foot into Extended Left Duck stance (remember to place your right heel down first).

At the same time swing your n u n c h a k u downwards to finish in the same position as movement number twentyone.

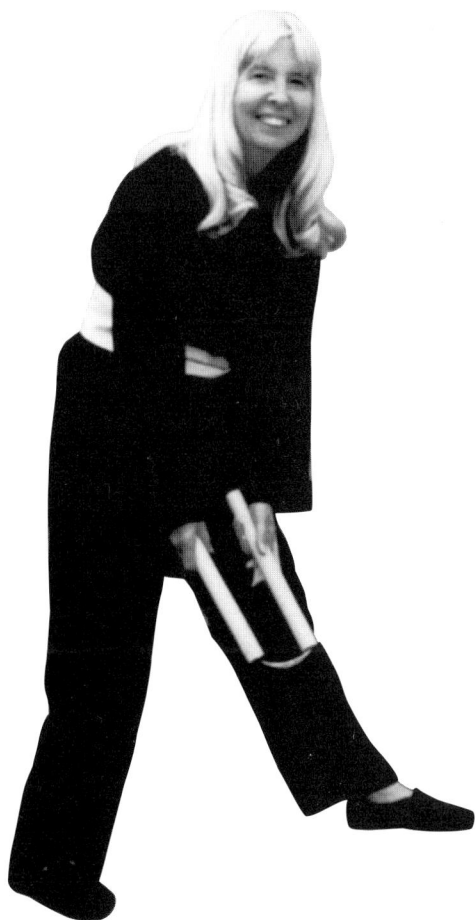

Number 123

From Extended Left Duck stance move your weight onto your left leg and raise your right leg into Right Crane stance (your right knee is bent, your right thigh is parallel to the floor).

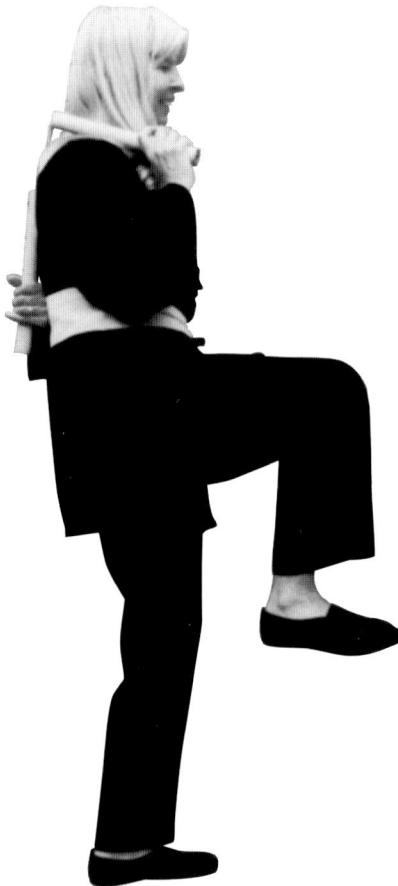

At the same time let go of your nunchaku with your left hand and swing the free end over your right shoulder, catching it with your left hand behind your back.

Number 124

From Right Crane stance turn one hundred and eighty degrees to your right into Right Dragon stance.

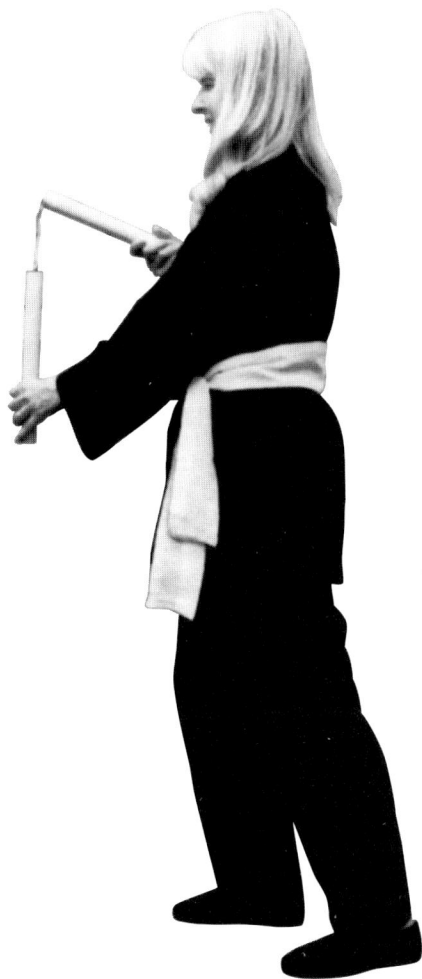

At the same time let go of your nunchaku with your left hand, your right arm extends forwards at shoulder height. Take hold of the free end with your left hand, finishing with your nunchaku in the same hand positions as they were in for movement number one hundred and twenty one.

LFA T'AI CHI NUNCHAKU

Number 125

From Right Dragon stance step behind with your right foot into Extended Left Duck stance. Remember to place your right heel down first.

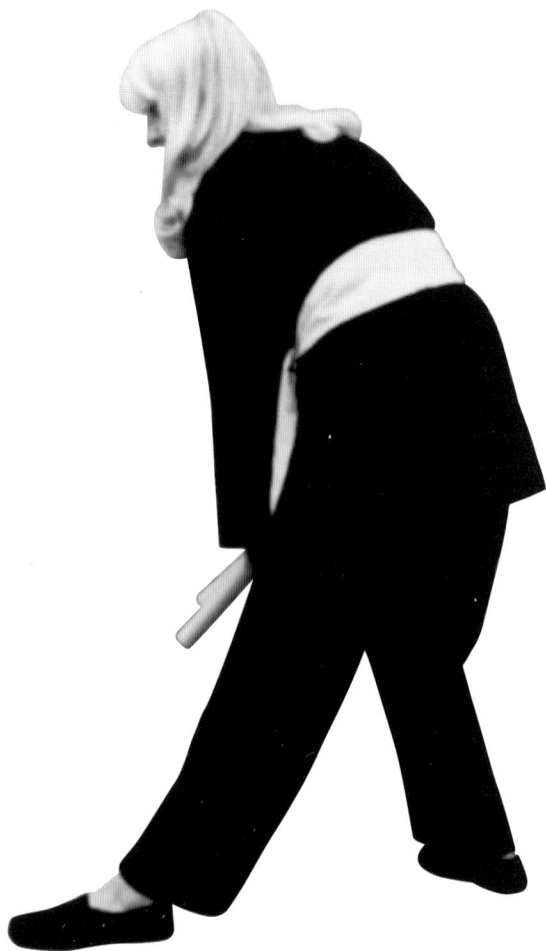

At the same time swing your nunchaku down into the same position as they were in for movement number one hundred and twenty two.

Number 126

From Extended Left Duck stance move your weight onto your left leg and raise your right leg into Right Crane stance (your right knee is bent, thigh parallel to the floor).

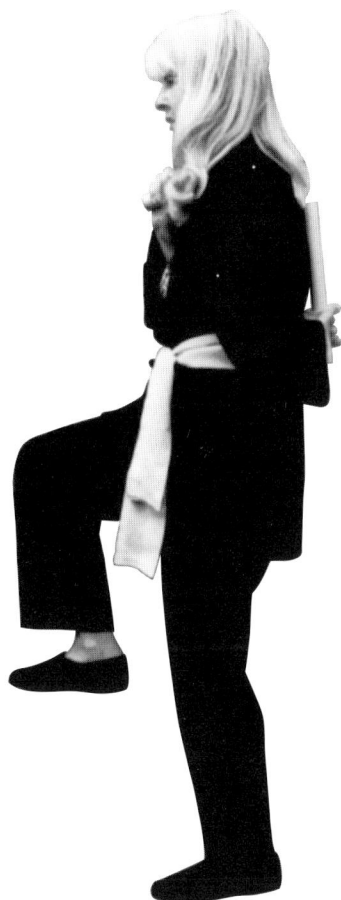

At the same time let go of your nunchaku with your left hand. Swing the free end over your right shoulder, catching it behind your back with your left hand.

Number 127

From Right Crane stance turn ninety degrees to your right into Left Scissors stance (both knees bent, the heel is raised on your left foot).

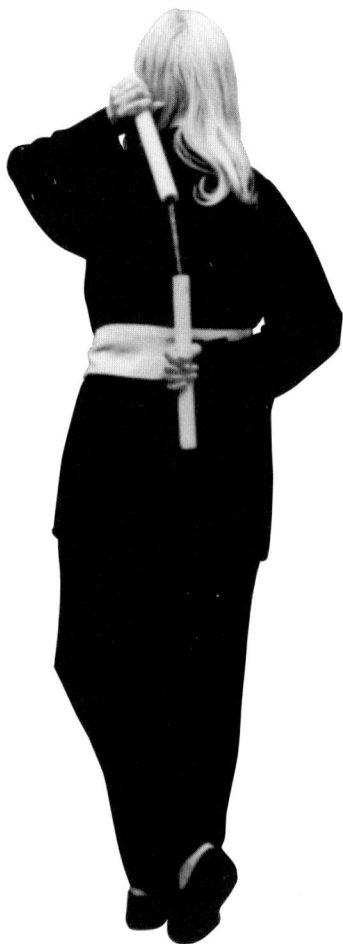

At the same time let go of your nunchaku with your right hand and swing the free end over your left shoulder, catching it with your right hand behind your back.

Number 128

From Left Scissors stance step sideways into Right Leopard stance (your right leg is bent and your left leg is straight).

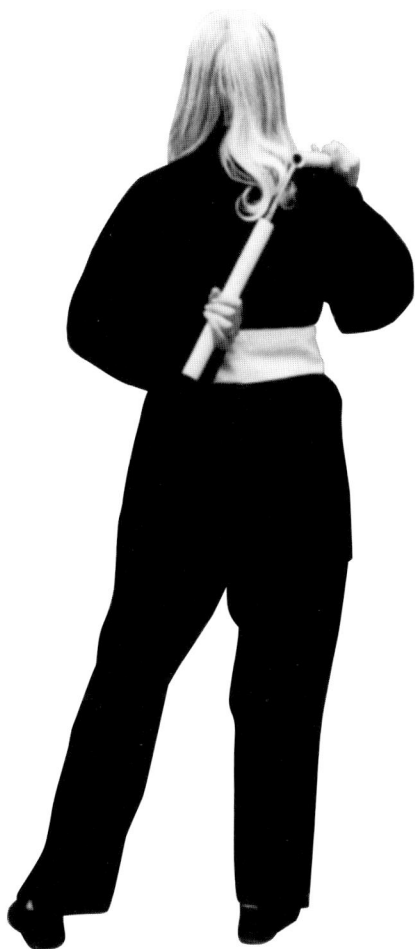

At the same time let go of your nunchaku with your left hand. Swing the free end over your right shoulder, catching it with your left hand behind your back.

Number 129

From into Right Leopard stance turn one hundred and eighty degrees to your right into Left Scissors stance.

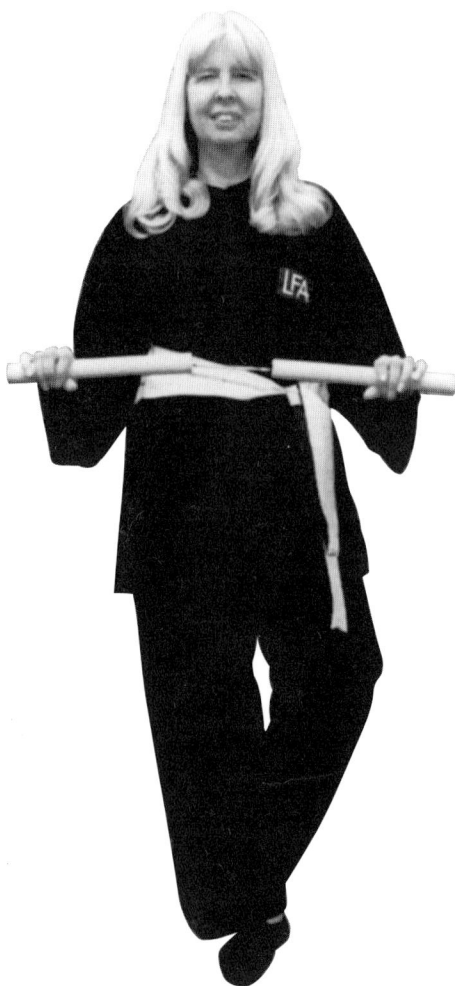

At the same time left go of your nunchaku with your right hand. Circle them around in front of your body e x c h a n g i n g them from your left hand to your right hand, then exchange them from your right hand to your left hand behind your back. Finally catch your nunchaku with your right hand. Your nunchaku finish horizontal at waist height).

Number 130

From Left Scissors stance turn ninety degrees to your left into Left Dragon stance.

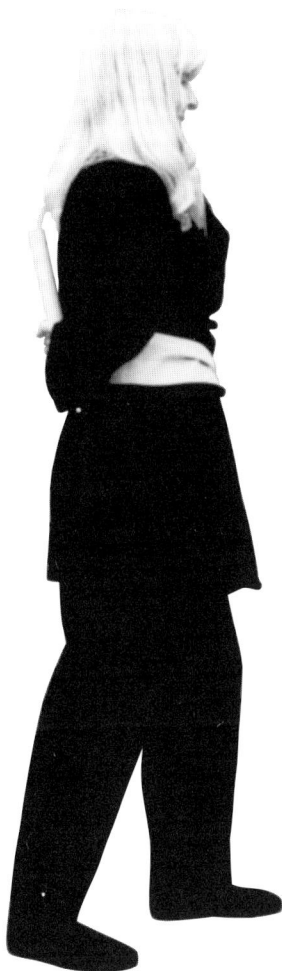

At the same time let go of your nunchaku with your right hand. Swing the free end of your nunchaku over your left shoulder, catching it behind your back with your right hand.

Number 131

From Left Dragon stance step forward into Right Dragon stance. Remember to apply the principles of the Taoist Walk.

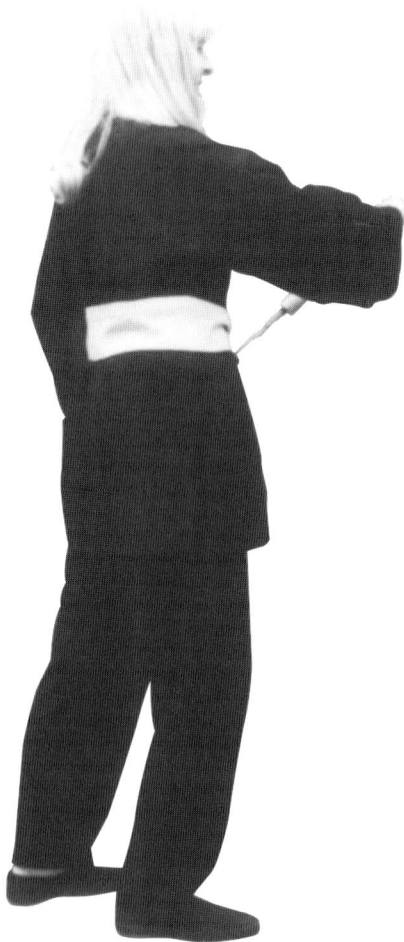

At the same time let go of your nunchaku with your left hand. With your right hand, pull your nunchaku round in front of your body and then swing the free end over to the left side of your body, catching it with your left hand Your nunchaku finish angled upwards from your left hip.

Number 132

From Right Dragon stance step through into Left Dragon stance. Remember to apply the principles of the Taoist Walk.

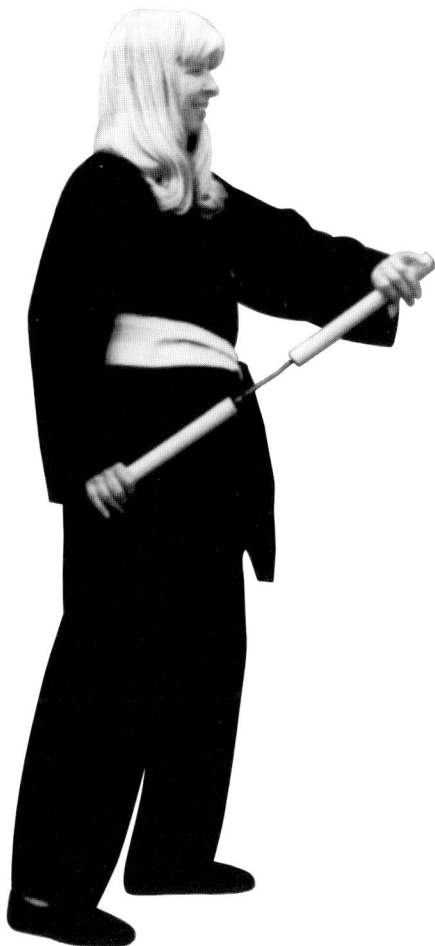

At the same time let go of your nunchaku with your right hand. Swing the free end of your nunchaku across to the right side of your body, catching it with your right hand. Your n u n c h a k u finish angled upwards from your right hip.

Number 133

From Left Dragon stance turn one hundred and eighty degrees to your left into Left Duck stance (right leg bent, left leg straight).

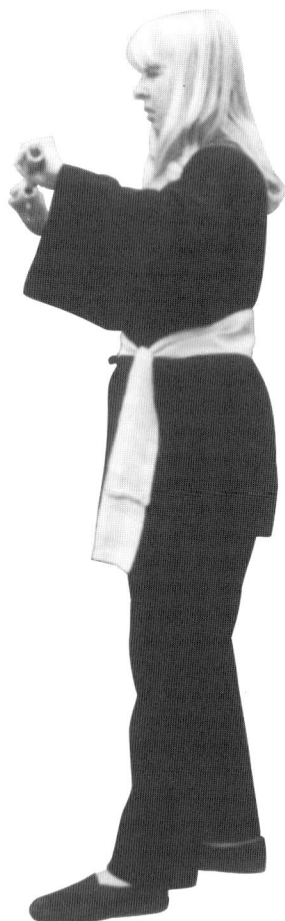

At the same time let go of your nunchaku with your left hand and catch the free end again with your left hand, (your nunchaku finish horizontal at shoulder height).

Number 134

From Left Duck stance step through into Right Cat stance (left knee bent, your heel is raised on your right foot).

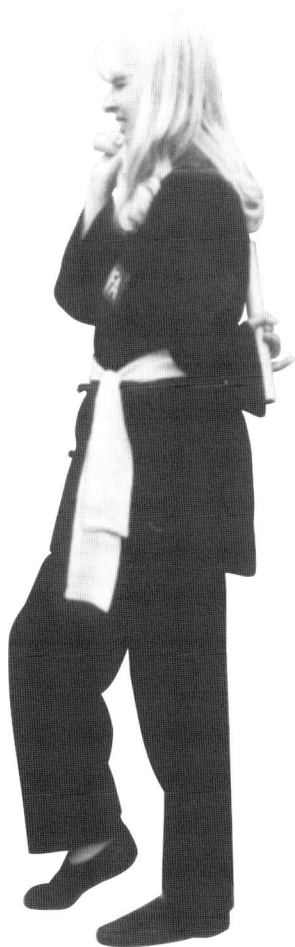

At the same time let go of your nunchaku with your left hand and swing the free end over your right shoulder, catching it with your left hand behind your back.

Number 135

From Right Cat stance place your right heel flat on the floor and raise your left leg into Left Crane stance (your left knee is bent, with your thigh parallel to the floor).

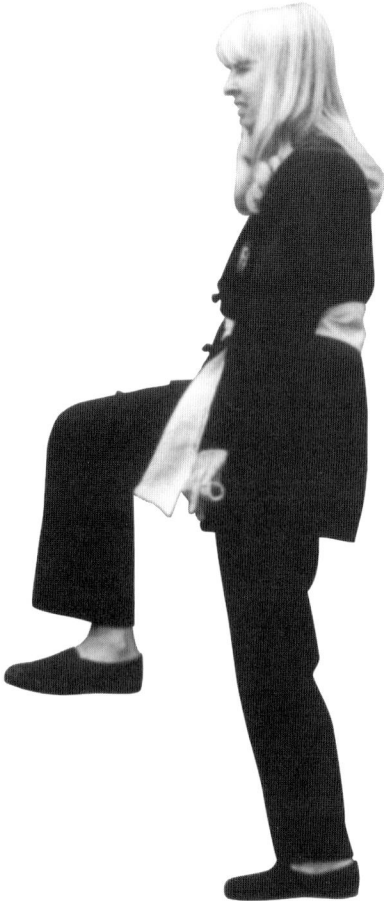

At the same time let go of your nunchaku with your right hand, swing the free end u n d e r n e a t h your left leg. Catch the free end of your nunchaku with your right hand.

Number 136

From Left Crane stance turn ninety degrees to your right into Right Chicken stance.

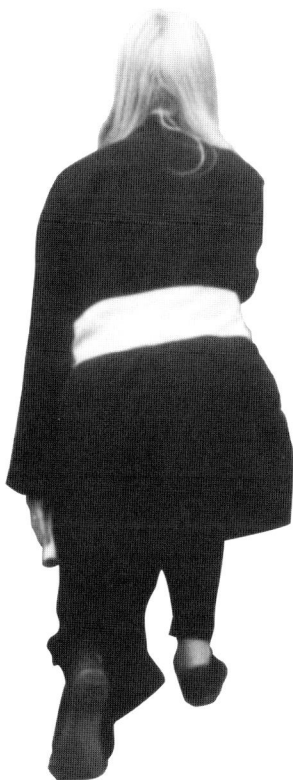

At the same time let go of your nunchaku with your left hand. Circle the free end of your nunchaku over the top and take hold of the free cnd with your left hand. Your left hand is by your left side.

Number 137

From Right Chicken stance step through into Left Dragon stance.

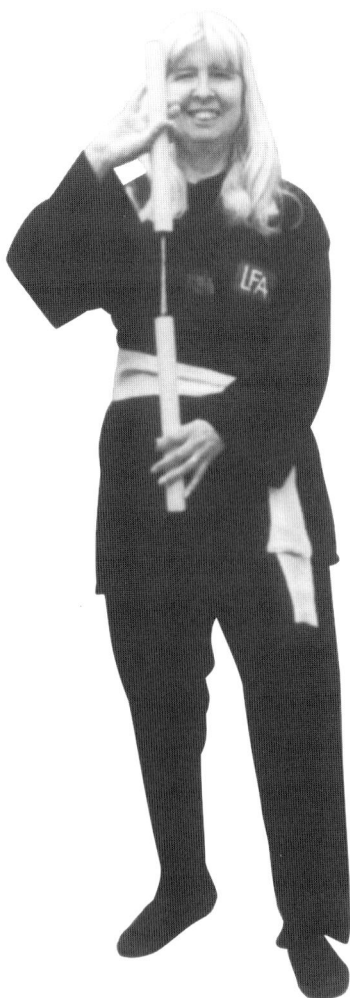

At the same time sweep your nunchaku forwards and upwards. Your nunchaku finish vertical (see photograph).

Note: the photograph shows the front view, but the actual stance is with the back facing the camera.

Number 138

From Left Dragon stance draw your left foot back into Bee stance (both heels together, toes pointing slightly outwards, both knees are bent).

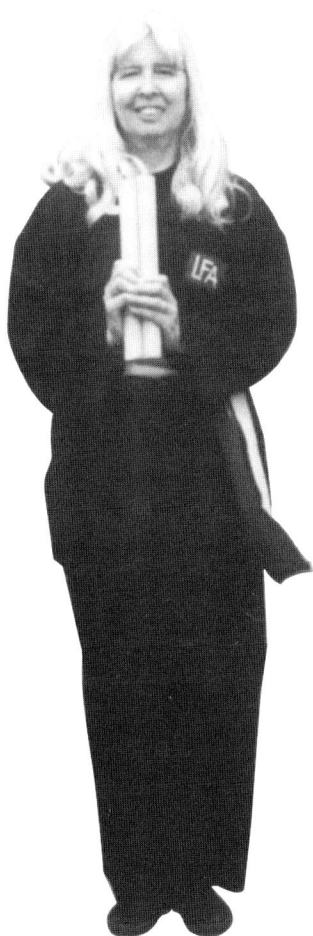

At the same time lower your right hand down so that both ends of your nunchaku are vertical (side by side).

Note: the photograph shows the front view, but the actual stance is with the back facing the camera.

Number 139

From Bee stance step sideways with your right foot into Right Leopard stance (right knee bent, left leg straight).

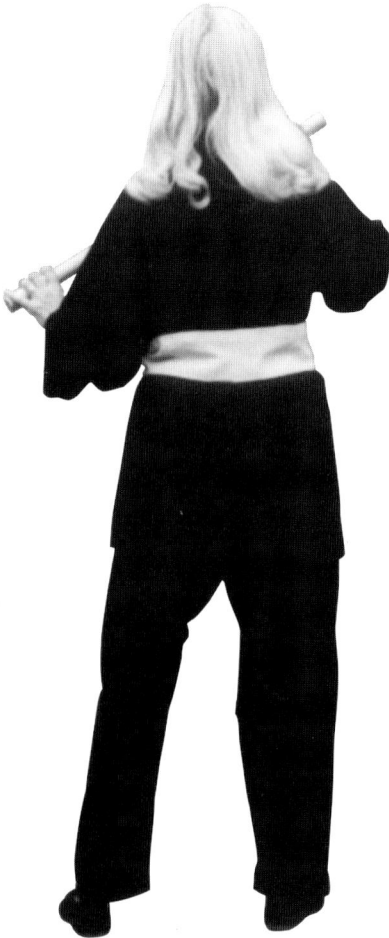

At the same time let go of your nunchaku with your left hand and complete one circle to the right. Catch the free end with your left hand. Your nunchaku finish angled downwards from right to left (see photograph).

Number 140

From Right Leopard stance cross your left foot behind your right leg into Left Scissors stance (both knees are bent, the heel is raised on your left foot).

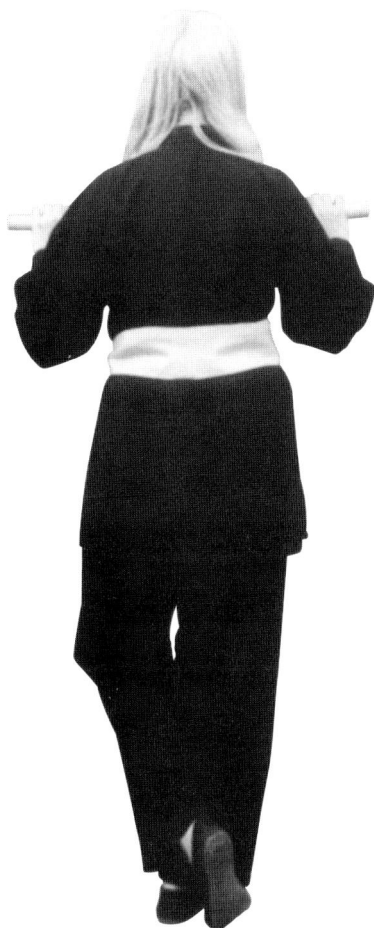

At the same time let go of your nunchaku with your left hand, circling them around your body. Exchange your nunchaku from your right hand to your left hand, and catch the free end with your right hand. Your nunchaku finish horizontal at shoulder height.

Number 141

From Left Scissors stance turn ninety degrees to your right into Right Dragon stance.

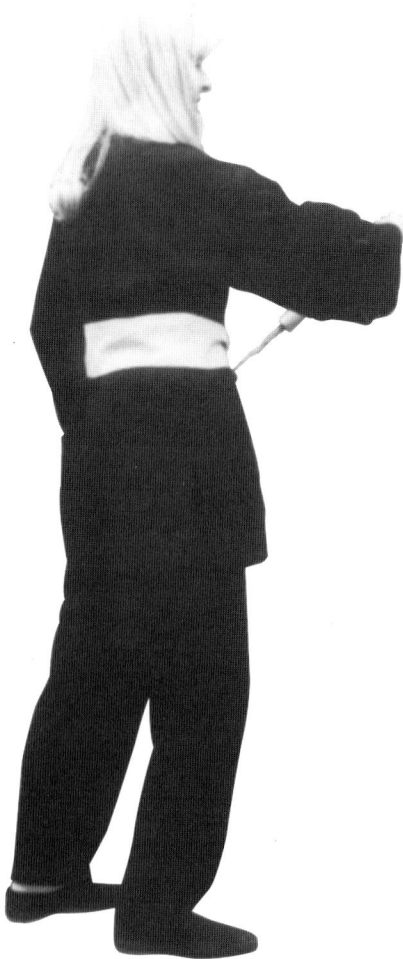

At the same time let go of your nunchaku with your left hand. Now flip the free end over (forwards) and catch it with your left hand at the left side of your body. Your nunchaku finish angled upwards from your left hip.

Number 142

From Right Dragon stance swing your left leg through into Left Dog stance.

At the same time sweep your right hand up to your right shoulder. Your nunchaku form a straight line.

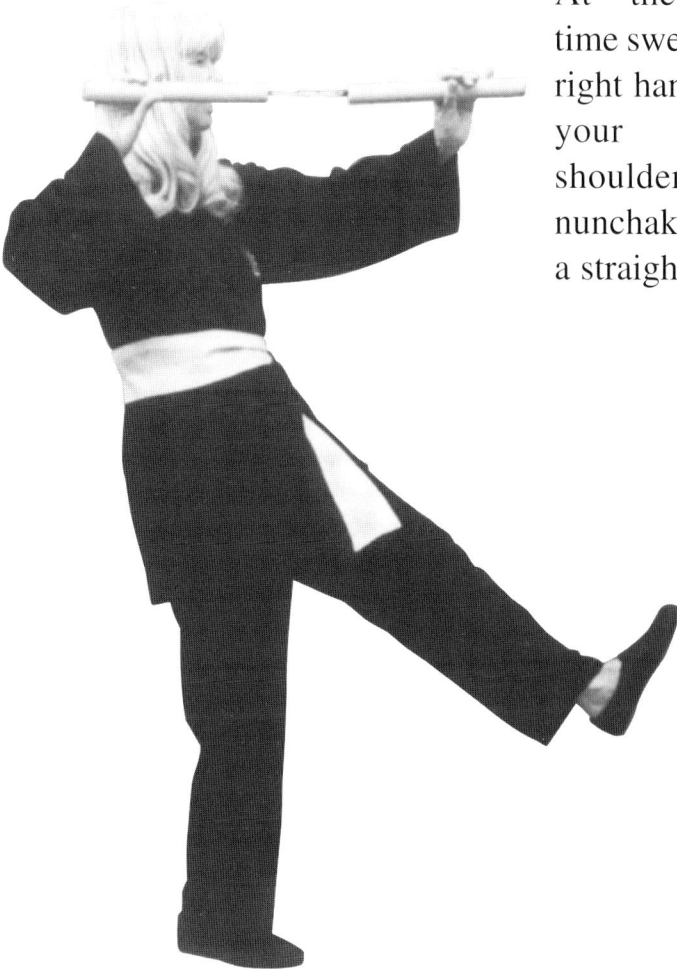

Number 143

From Left Dog stance step through into Left Dragon stance.

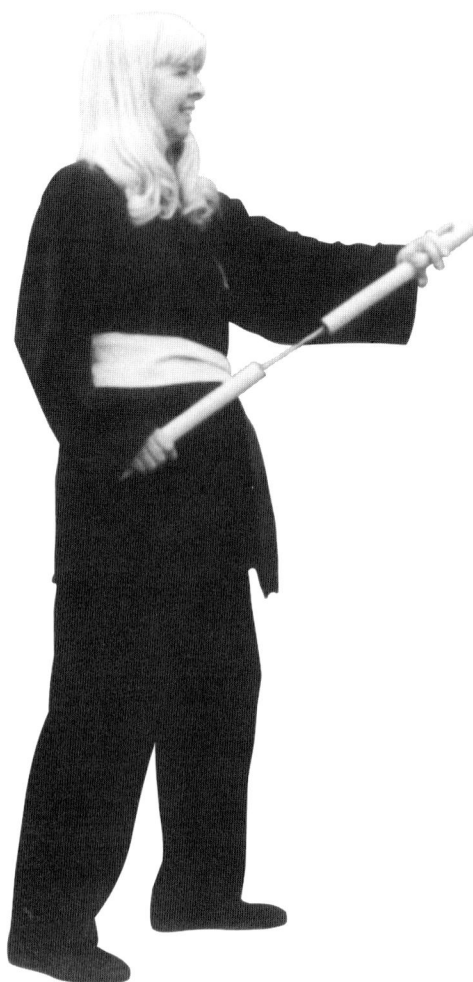

At the same time let go of your nunchaku with your right hand. Flip the free end over (forwards) and catch it with your right hand at the right side of your body. Your nunchaku finish angled upwards from your right hip.

Number 144

From Left Dragon stance step behind with your left foot into Right Duck stance (left leg bent, your right leg is straight).

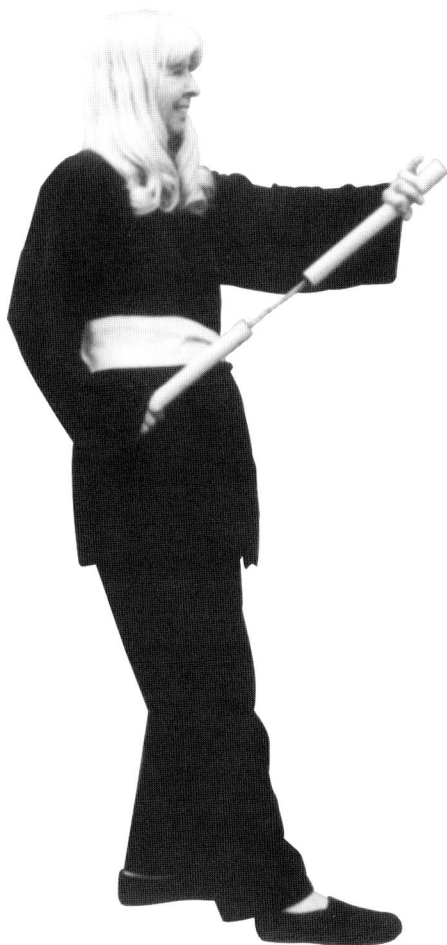

At the same time let go of your nunchaku with your left hand. Now circle your right arm backwards (flipping the free end of your nunchaku over, then forwards) catching the free end with your left hand. Your nunchaku finish angled upwards from your right hip.

Number 145

From Right Duck stance step behind with your right foot into Left Duck stance (right leg bent, your left leg is straight).

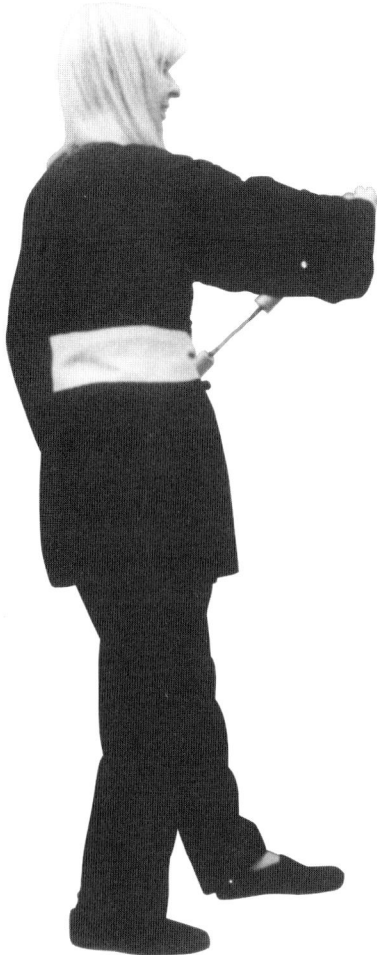

At the same time let go of your nunchaku with your right hand. Now circle your left arm backwards (flipping the free end of your nunchaku over and then u p w a r d s) finally catching it with your right hand. Your nunchaku finish angled upwards from your left hip.

Number 146

From Left Duck stance turn ninety degrees to your left into Right Scissors (both knees bent, the heel is raised on your right foot).

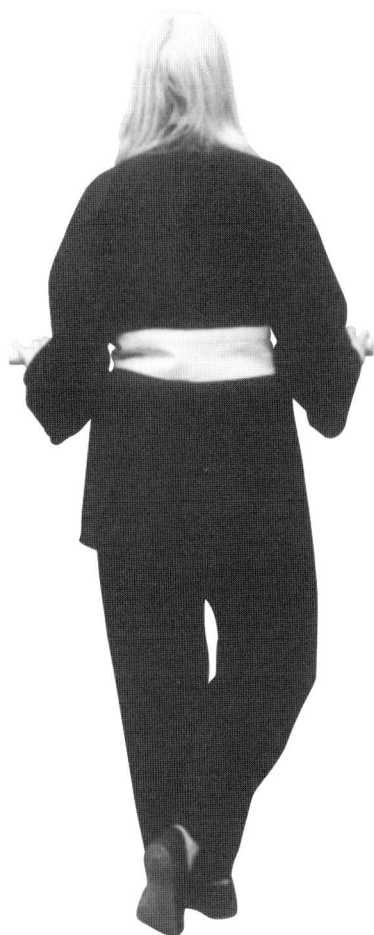

At the same time your nunchaku move to the horizontal position at waist height.

Number 147

From Right Scissors stance step sideways into Left Leopard stance (left knee bent, your right leg is straight).

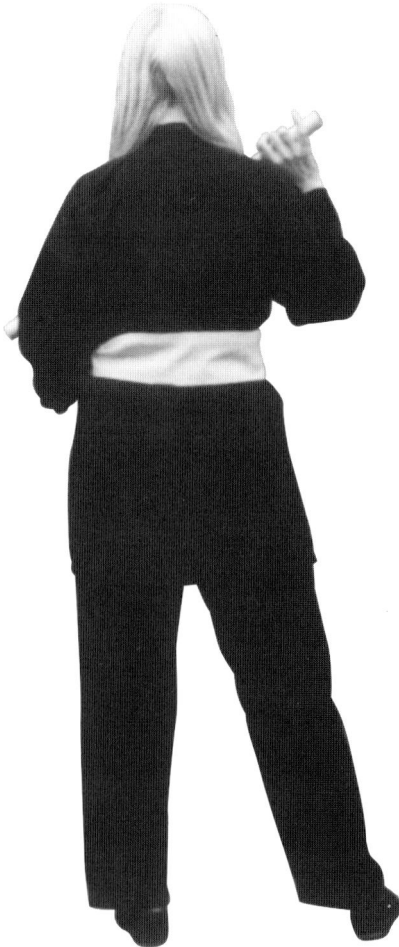

At the same time let go of your nunchaku with your left hand. Circle the free end to your right catching it with your left hand, to finish with your nunchaku angled downwards from right to left.

Number 148

From Left Leopard stance turn one hundred and eighty degrees to your right into Left Scissors stance (both knees bent, the heel is raised on your left foot).

At the same time move your nunchaku to the horizontal position at waist height.

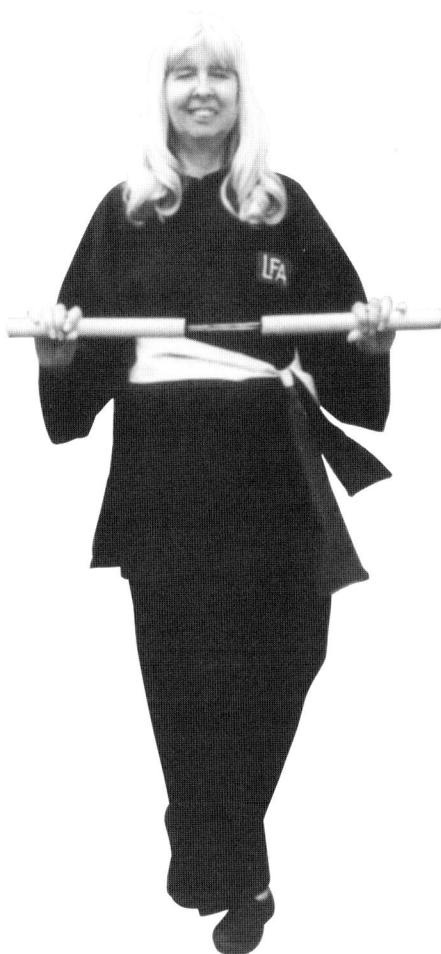

Number 149

From Left Scissors stance step sideways into Left Leopard stance (left knee bent, your right leg is straight).

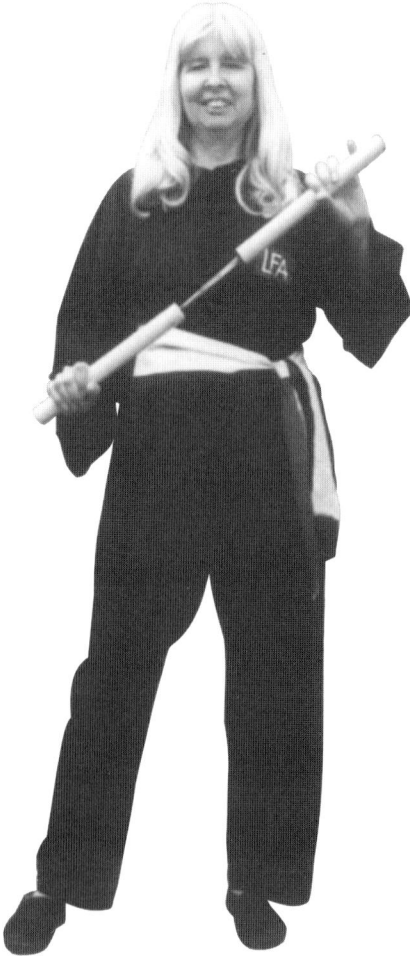

At the same time move your left hand to your left shoulder and your right hand to your right hip.

Number 150

From Left Leopard stance draw your left foot into Eagle stance (both heels together, your toes are pointing slightly outwards).

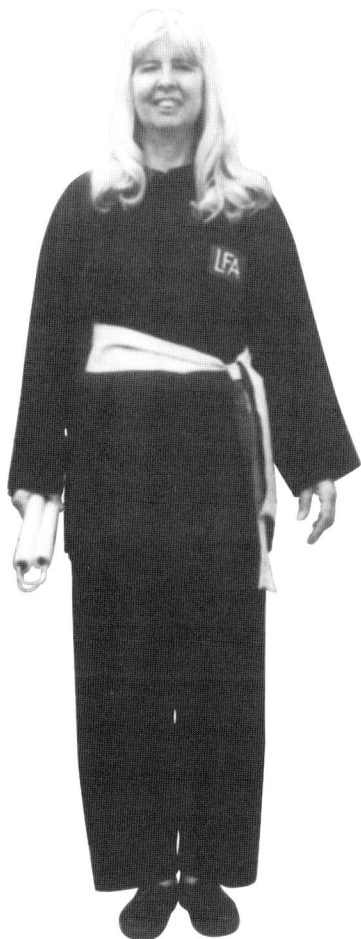

At the same time place both ends of your nunchaku in your right hand. Both arms finish by your sides.

The LFA T'ai Chi Nunchaku Set is for everyone. This book is more than a beginners' guide because for the first time in 3000 years, the first 150 movements of our Nunchaku set are in print for the benefit of the people in the West. The LFA retain full copyright on the movements in this book as they have not previously been available to the public.

To find the inner depth within the movements, you may wish to train with us at our ever growing number of LFA classes and day courses as shown on our Website.

I hope you have enjoyed learning the first one hundred and fifty movements of our Nunchaku Set and look forward to meeting you in our classes and on our courses.

We intend to publish the remainder of the movements in a subsequent book in the not too distant future. May you continue to enjoy your journey with the Lee Family Arts.

LFA T'AI CHI NUNCHAKU

Notes

LFA T'AI CHI NUNCHAKU

Notes